Time for Dementia

A collection of writings on the meanings of time and dementia

Time is not a length of calico.
Time is a mist that never stops moving.
– from *I saw Ramallah,* by Mourid Barghouti

Edited by Jane Gilliard & Mary Marshall
Illustrated by James McKillop

HAWKER PUBLICATIONS

Time for Dementia

First published in 2010 by
Hawker Publications Ltd,
Culvert House, Culvert Road,
London SW11 5DH
Tel: 020 7720 2108
www.careinfo.org

British Library Cataloguing in Publication Data
A catalogue record for this book is available from the British Library

ISBN 9781874790921

Designed and copy edited by Andrew Chapman, www.awrc.co.uk and Sue Benson
Set in Baskerville and Futura

Printed and bound in Great Britain by Information Press Ltd, Oxford

Cover and section introduction photographs by James McKillop.
These photographs were first published by the Dementia Services Development Centre,
Stirling University in *Opening Shutters, Opening Minds* by James McKillop, 2003.
We are grateful for their permission to use the photographs in this book.
For permission to reproduce contact dementia@stir.ac.uk.

We also acknowledge and thank Roger McGough and Viking for permission
to publish the poem on page 111.

Hawker Publications publishes the *Journal of Dementia Care* and *Caring Times*.

Contents

Introduction

Jane Gilliard & Mary Marshall

Professor Jane Gilliard is a social worker who has worked in dementia care for over 25 years. She established Dementia Voice, the dementia services development centre for south west England and was its Director from 1997 to 2005. She was the Chair of the National Network of Dementia Services Development Centres and has been involved in many key national working groups in dementia care. Jane was a member of the NICE/SCIE Dementia Guideline Development Group and the Working Group which developed the National Dementia Strategy. She is now the National Programme Manager for supporting the implementation of the strategy. Jane is a Visiting Professor at the University of the West of England, Bristol.

Mary Marshall is Emeritus Professor at the University of Stirling where she was the Director of the Dementia Services Development Centre until 2005. She has worked with older people as a social worker, researcher, campaigner and manager. She is now a sessional inspector with the Social Work Inspection Agency and she writes and lectures on dementia care.

The idea for this collection of writings arose from a conversation between Jane and Chris Sherratt when both were working for Dementia Voice, the dementia services development centre for south west England. Chris noticed that care staff often commented that they had insufficient time simply to be with people with dementia. Their days were taken up with practical tasks; management practices often meant they were made to feel as if they were wasting time if they simply sat with residents; and the organisational culture required them to be continually busy. He reflected that the word 'time' comes up frequently and that there must be many uses of the word throughout dementia care.

The idea for the book was born and it really resonated with Mary and subsequently with everyone we asked to contribute. We use the word all the time, yet rarely stop to appreciate the way we use it. So often we use it negatively. Perhaps if we were more sensitive to this we might seek to understand the reasons.

When we say we do not have time for 'person centred care', or "spending time talking to people with dementia" or "enabling them to do things for themselves even though it takes longer" – what are we really saying? Are we saying that spending time with a person with dementia has less value than a staff meeting for example, or tidying up? Time is the currency of dementia care; we spend it on what we value most.

Perhaps we are not in control of our time; someone else tells us what to do. They might value a tidy lounge more highly than a personal interaction, or they might want everyone up and dressed by a certain time. This can be very demoralising to staff with knowledge and expertise in relating to people with dementia and their carers.

The phrase "time is money" can be true in dementia care since staff costs are the greatest part of any budget. The person responsible for the budget may have priorities that are not about communication and personal interaction. For them the fact that people with dementia take longer may be something they prefer to ignore. Their priorities may be about the number of assessments, the extra days in a hospital bed, or the number of people visited.

Where does this come from? Is it pressure from within the organisation, or outside it? Is

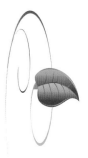

it a cultural perspective that misunderstands dementia and percolates through our practices?

People working in health and social care in the UK in the first decade of the 21st century tend to be hyper-time-conscious. This is in spite of the number of labour-saving devices we have in our homes and offices. Every day is filled to the brim. Blackberries and mobile phones are never switched off; a broken watch is a major handicap; and losing a printed or electronic diary is catastrophic. Hours are spent each day planning the future. Time management is rarely achieved. We always seem to be running late. Catching planes and trains imposes time anxiety for hours before they leave.

On the other hand, people who are not working lose this day-by-day, hour-by-hour awareness of time to some extent. Does the date matter if you have no commitments? People with dementia often have no need to know the time and date, yet their dementia is often assessed by their ability or inability to relate to time. They are surrounded by professionals for whom it is vital. In our hyper-time-conscious world, this indifference to time puts them speedily into the category of 'other' – a parallel and very different universe. They no longer fit into the majority world, which is the one, generally speaking, which makes the most important decisions.

There is no denying that people with dementia can take longer. They can take longer to wash, dress, eat and so on, as well as to collect their thoughts and communicate. From their point of view, the rushing about that goes on all around them can be very alarming and often undermines their confidence. For example, the speedy world of the acute hospital ward can be especially disabling. Making time for a person who takes longer can be a real nuisance to someone in a hurry. People with dementia thereby can make the lives of those around them problematic – routines are undermined, and delays get into the system. The upshot can be that things are done 'to' people with dementia because it is quicker. Meaningful and personal conversations are often avoided. This is, of course, easier if you believe that people with dementia have nothing to say which is meaningful.

You may be puzzled that this book begins with such an outpouring of negativity. We consider it important to confront this so that we are all clear about the extent of negative thinking around this word 'time'. We can use the word without appreciating this negative thinking and without dealing with the issues behind it. We want to make it clear that we believe the problem lies with the non-dementia world. It is almost a culture clash between the hyper-time-conscious world and people for whom time is unimportant. The former, of course, has the power.

People with dementia have less time than the rest of us for all the gifts they bring to the world: their ability to be true to their feelings, to be really in the moment, often to be creative, to demonstrate courage in the face of one of life's greatest possible challenges and so on. For them time is running out quickly and those of us without dementia need to seize the time whenever we can.

This book is not a major academic text on the nature of time, time and older people or time and dementia of which there are several (examples listed below). Instead it is an attempt to blow the word 'time' out of the water, to make us stop and think about it and to make decisions to be more positive. This may require a change of priorities, or processes. It may require the non-dementia world to slow down: to be in the moment.

Baars J, Visser H (eds) (2007) *Aging and Time: Multidisciplinary Perspectives*. Baywood, Amityville, New York.
Goodin RE, Rice JM, Parpo A, Eriksson L (2008) *Discretionary Time, A new measure of freedom*. Cambridge University Press, Cambridge.
Klein S (2008) *Time: a user's guide*. Penguin Books, London.
McFadden S, Atchley RC (eds) (2001) *Aging and the meaning of time*. Springer Publishing Company, New York.

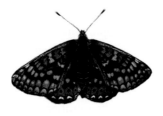

Making this book

This book is an anthology of pieces written by people we highly respect, who work in the field of dementia care. We asked for anything between 200 and 1,000 words in prose or poems.

We were surprised and delighted with the responses – poetic writings from academic staff; personal stories from professional colleagues; moving contributions from people with dementia and their carers. We have been enchanted with the contributions, which led us to divide the book loosely into sections for ease of access.

We begin with some reflections on the meaning of the word 'time' itself. Then we have a set of contributions on the need to make time in busy worlds of work. Some pieces were very clearly about clocks. The moving section on time to love is about relationships within couples and families. The contributions are mainly written by relatives of someone with dementia.

Being in the moment is the key challenge for dementia care, so there is a large section on this. Night time is a time needing greater attention and we were pleased that several contributors addressed this. We expected more about both past times and pastimes; these are brief but important sections, and the topics come up in other sections too. We conclude with a section on making the best use of time, which also includes our reflections on the whole set of contributions.

Terminology

We have sought to achieve consistency in the use of certain key words. We have used the word 'carer' to refer to family and friends of people with dementia; and we have used the term 'care staff' or 'care worker' to refer to paid staff. Throughout we have tried to refer to 'people with dementia' because we think the term 'sufferer' is unhelpful, but there are a small number of occasions where people with dementia have used the word 'sufferer' themselves and in this case we have left the word as it stands. We have also mostly avoided words like 'patient', 'client' or 'service user' except where the writing refers to a particular care setting where one of these words is applicable.

Where there are acronyms, we have spelt out their meaning in full or in a footnote.

There are some culturally specific terms. In Australia, for example, they have a system of dementia hostels – a facility with no direct comparison in the UK. Dementia hostels offer a service somewhere between the UK care home and sheltered housing models.

Acknowledgements

We would like formally to thank all our contributors who took our request with such seriousness and gave us such thoughtful contributions. We are also grateful to Chris Sherratt who had the original idea for this book, and encouraged us to do it. Sue Benson and Richard Hawkins saw the point of the book and agreed to publish it which gave us the push we needed to deliver it. James McKillop provided the photographs as well as a written contribution.

Quotations about time are interspersed through the book. Rosas Mitchell found us the lines by Mourid Barghouti, quoted on the title page. John Killick suggested the quotation from Granta on page 10. Claire Craig asked a group of residents in a Sheffield care home what time meant to them, and their responses are shared on page 54. We are very grateful to Roger McGough for permission to reprint part of his poem *Hard Times* on page 111.

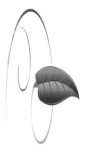

Dedication

To everyone in dementia care, in the hope that we can all make more time to enjoy the all too brief opportunities to be in the moment with people with dementia and to learn from people with dementia about how this can be achieved.

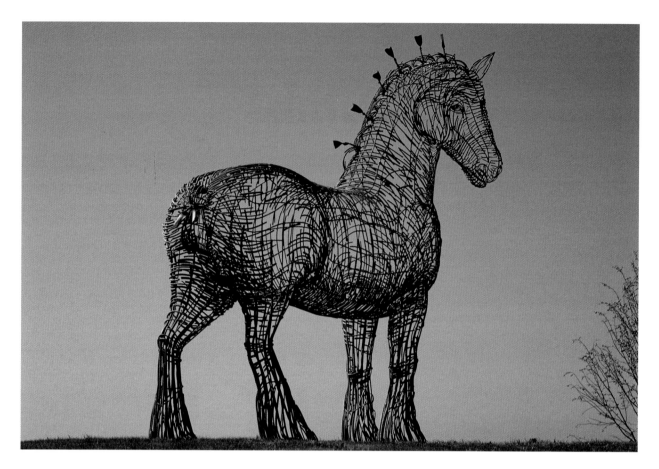

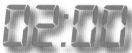

The meaning of time

Crumbs

Anon

Tin of biscuits
In my mouth there are crumbs
Means I must have had one - again
Escaping me

Losing seconds
Outstripping
Self
Scary

Time doesn't click on and on at the stroke. It comes and goes in waves and folds like water; it flutters and sifts like dust, rises, billows, falls back on itself. When a wave breaks the water is not moving. The swell has travelled great distances but only the energy is moving, not the water. Perhaps time moves through us and not us through it.
Tim Winton
From 'Aquifer' Granta 70 Australia (2000) p.52

02:02

Time passage

John Keady

John Keady is Professor of Older People's Mental Health Nursing, a joint appointment between the University of Manchester and the Greater Manchester West Mental Health NHS Foundation Trust. He is founding and co-editor of 'Dementia: The International Journal of Social Research and Practice', a quarterly Sage journal first published in February 2002.

"I don't see time the way you do." Those words haunt me and I have long reflected upon their meaning. The context of their speaking is a little easier to describe. They were shared during an interview I was conducting with a widowed 62-year-old man who was living alone with his Alzheimer's disease. I will call him Steven. I was at Steven's home to discuss how he lived his life day by day now that he spent most of his waking moments on his own. The first three questions on my interview schedule were:

- 'How do you start each day?'
- 'What are the most important times of your day?'
- 'What are the main challenges that you face?'

We were sitting together in Steven's lounge surrounded by the clutter of his life. Unopened mail. Newspapers strewn across the floor. Scribbled 'Post it' notes glued onto doorframes: 'DON'T FORGET' their bold, headline message. The clock on the mantelpiece was motionless, its hands stuck on the numbers 8 and 4. I noticed the family photograph next to the clock. It had fallen. I asked if I could pick it up and Steven gave me his permission. I looked at the faded colours on the photograph. Smiling faces, a family group, stared back at me. Steven looked much younger. I returned the photograph to its precarious position; it wouldn't be too long until it fell again. The sun lit up the curtainless room. It was daytime. It was summertime. The sun brought warmth. The noise of traffic and human voices filtered into our private space through an open window.

I started to ask my questions.

Steven was patient and initially struggled for words to describe his feeling and thoughts about how he started each day. I was grateful for his words. I then asked my second question, the one with the word 'time' in it. "I don't see time the way you do," came the reply.

I was taken aback by this sudden insight into Steven's world. I asked Steven what he meant by those words. "Everything." "What do you mean by everything Steven?" After a slight hesitation, he replied:

"I don't see time the way you see time. I live it. Sometimes it goes quickly. Sometimes it goes slowly. Sometimes it just goes and then I see the dark and feel the cold. Time passes. Time passage. You're living there now. A time passage. I will forget you."

I had my answer.

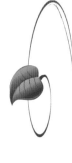

02:03

Time, dementia and general practice

Steve Iliffe

Professor Steve Iliffe is an academic general practitioner who has worked in a large socially diverse inner-city group practice in NW London for 30 years. He is co-director (with Professor Ann Bowling) of the Centre for Ageing Population Studies in the Department of Primary Care and Population Sciences at University College London. He is Associate Director for the UK national co-ordinating centre for Dementias & Neurodegenerative Diseases Research Networks (DeNDRoN), was a member of the NICE dementia guidelines development group from 2004 to 2006, and also of the Age Concern Inquiry into Mental Health and Well-being in Later Life, in 2006.

In general practice there seems to be too little time for dementia. Some general practitioners feel profoundly unskilled in dealing with the problems that dementia syndromes create (Iliffe *et al* 2006). They struggle with the difficulties of diagnosis, find it hard to respond to behavioural and psychological symptoms, and avoid caring for people with dementia in care homes, at the end of their lives. Transfer of responsibility for the person with dementia occurs rapidly – *in no time* – with the hope that specialist services will become the main source of support for the individual and their family. These doctors emphasise the unpredictable demands that they face, the heavy and growing workload of general practice, their struggle to *organise time* effectively, and the difficulty of coping with *competing demands on time* (Pritchard 1992).

Those general practitioners who accept a role in working with a person with dementia and their families or carers still worry about time. They know that reaching the diagnosis always *takes time*. In the beginning the changes that occur in thinking, memory or behaviour are small things, easily attributed to ageing – *the passage of time* –and appear through the personality of the individual. Suspicions grow *over time* into concerns, and concerns have to be explored in a *timely* way – not so fast that the person with dementia is hurried onto an escalator of disablement, but not so slowly that opportunities to understand or act are missed, and *time wasted* (De Lepeleire *et al* 1994). These doctors know that they have *plenty of time*, that they can

wait and see, talk with the person again, and see family members and others who can describe the *timescale* of the individual's change. They can also prepare the person with suspected dementia for the *time-consuming* psychological tests that are carried out in the memory clinic. Nevertheless they still feel *time-pressures* acutely, wondering whether they can fit a cognitive function test into a consultation; one of the curiosities of dementia research is the pursuit of the *brief* screening test.

People with dementia have *limited time*. They can become *disoriented in time*, and have no control over the timescale of the disease, for as yet the course of dementia syndromes cannot be modified. Services and support for people with dementia are complex and sometimes inconsistent; it can take *so much time* to sort them out that a new job can be created to *make time*: the dementia care co-ordinator.

Time and power are disconnected (Frankenberg 1992). The most powerful people in dementia care are 10-minute people, the doctors who interpret test results and make decisions. They may not take time to listen to their patients as much as *take a history*. The next most powerful are nurses or social workers, who may be two-hour people (at least sometimes). Family members and friends who do the bulk of the caring are 12- to 24-hour people, but they often have the least formal control over what happens, and frequently *their time is not their own*.

The tragic, because inevitable, contradiction of modern, scientific medicine is that its application so often depends on the timescale of disease, while its efficacy lies in the timescale of illness (Frankenberg 1992). To analyse and treat disease the doctor must step back from the patient's subjective world and place them on the conveyor belt of diagnosis, which moves *at its own pace*. However, to really help the person after the diagnostic process is complete, the doctor needs to meet them *in their own time*, within their individual experience of illness. General practitioners move between the two tasks, sometimes with discomfort and difficulty. It is no surprise that specialists criticise them for their *tardiness* in reaching diagnoses that are obvious enough when seen from a distance.

This contradiction may not be resolvable, but it can be attenuated. Pritchard describes the deliberate attempt to understand the patient's appreciation of time as *'time empathy'* (an alternative to *time management*, perhaps). General practitioners can sidestep taking a history and instead *take a present* of the person's social and psychological being, and their becoming. Most important of all, 12- to 24-hour people can be *given time* to tell their side of the story, and the 10-minute people can learn to take *time out* to explain themselves.

Iliffe S, Wilcock J, Haworth D (2006) Obstacles to shared care for patients with dementia: a qualitative study. *Family Practice* doi:1093/fampra/cmi116.

Pritchard P (1992) Doctors, Patients & Time in Frankenberg R (ed) *Time Health & Medicine*. Sage, London.

De Lepeleire J, Heyrman J, Buntinx F (1998). The early diagnosis of dementia: triggers, early signs and luxating events. *Family Practice* 15: 431-436.

Frankenberg R (1992) 'Your time or mine?': temporal contradictions of biomedical practice in Frankenberg R (ed) *Time Health & Medicine*. Sage, London.

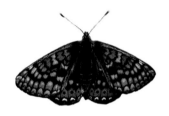

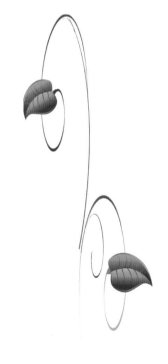

Time on our side?

Joan Maizels

Joan Maizels was born in London in 1918, the youngest of five children. Following her marriage during the war, she became an acclaimed social science researcher, committed feminist and political activist, publishing a number of academic and polemic books. On retirement, she took up poetry, resumed her childhood love of playing the piano, and embarked on an OU degree in the arts, followed by an MA in Women's Studies, from which she graduated at the age of 77. She began developing Alzheimer's in her early 80s and at age 88 chose to live in a Sunrise Reminiscence Community, in which she has continued her love of reading, observing human interactions, and building warm relationships. She wrote this poem before she developed dementia. It comes from *Stepping Gently: Poems by Joan Maizels*, Bumblebee Press, Edinburgh 1998.

Time is a woman
with a hone in her hand
who smiles and spits
as she sharpens her wits
and counts the hours.

Time is a woman
with her fingers on the strings
as she plucks and plays
she counts the days
and calls the tune.

Time is a woman
who's smashed her crystal ball
she beats a drum
for things to come
and counts her dues.

02:05

Away and somewhere else

John Killick

John Killick is a writer, researcher and broadcaster. His most recent publication is *Dementia Diary: Poetry and Prose*. His website is: www.dementiapositive.co.uk.

For most of us time is a significant concept, and one which can, if we do not guard against it, come to dominate our lives. The days of the week, months of the year, years of our span, are markers of achievement or failure to take our opportunities. We look forward, and we look back, and what happened in the past is often allowed to influence what will occur in the future.

How is this capacity affected by the disability of dementia? Quite profoundly, it seems. Memory loss and failing intellectual powers create gaps and confusions which inhibit the processes of taking stock and anticipation. Experience increasingly becomes a matter of isolated perceptions – isolated both from each other and from the interpretative faculty which would enable them to be set in a context. This state of arrested perception is well characterised in a line from the poet Louis MacNeice:

Time was away and somewhere else.

Of course this does not mean that the person has gone away, as is often claimed of individuals with the condition, only that a certain faculty is no longer present. This can prove both a relief and a release. The place people are inhabiting may be available to, but neglected by, the rest of us. It can lead to an intensity of appreciation of the moment, as in this celebration of the grounds of a care home in the words of one of its residents:

It's a wonderful setting,
this whole melting scene.
Is it opening or seizing?
The view: it's got the ring of expand.

Or the enhanced sense of wonder encapsulated in the following lines from a poem by another woman:

There's beauty in everything
if you look for it:
the sky from the skylight
in colours or not.
It depends on your mood.

Oh I went to look up in the sky
and saw it shining there
and said "That is Life."

I have tried to express something of the challenge and the opportunity of the consequences of this changed concept of time in my own 'Dementia Haiku':

This gift I bring you,
please handle it carefully:
it is the present.

Louis Macneice (2001) *Selected Poems*. Edited Michael Longley. Faber, London.
The two poems by people with dementia quoted from, as well as my own 'Dementia Haiku', are to be found in my book: Killick J (2008) *Dementia Diary*. Hawker Publications, London.

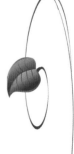

Reflections on the meaning of time in dementia care

Louise Skrypnuik

Louise is undertaking a Masters in Occupational Therapy at Curtin University, Australia having previously worked in the business sector. She has a BA in international business. One of her Masters placements was with the Mary Chester Centre, a dementia-specific day respite centre run by AAWA (Alzheimers Australia, Western Australia) where she and a fellow student facilitated a small group of men who reflected on what time meant to them using prompts such as photographs and poems.

Jim

Lithe like a greyhound, softly spoken and our day centre 'volunteer'. Never wanting to be seen to be sitting down on the job, he prefers to stand and is always willing to give us a hand.

Quick with the witty one-liners is 74-year-old Jim, and this is what I was expecting when I asked him, "What does time mean to you?" Instead he replied: "Time is not very easy to analyse…Time is fluid…Time is precious." These words from Jim offer a powerful insight.

Tom

"Daisy, Daisy give me your answer do." This is the melody I associate with Tom. He is 80 years of age and looks remarkable young, with his gentle blue eyes and broad smile. He often bursts into song: no occasion is needed. Singing is what he does. He speaks with a strong Geordie accent and is proud of his roots. Time to Tom is constant. "Time waits for no man," he tells me and "Everybody has to have time". He shares with me: "When my wife was alive, there were plenty of happy times," and sums up his feelings of time by stating "I believe time is life".

David

A university lecturer in his day, David is a smartly dressed man who enters the day centre using a wheeled walker with a briefcase placed on the seat. He is highly intelligent and on a good day he shares his brilliance with those who are around him. David has Lewy body dementia and is acutely insightful of his condition.

When asked how he spends his time, he looks me in the eye and tells me that he tries "to maintain a balance, which means I do not stress myself and my solution is sleep, this combats my version of dementia". He adds: "I sleep because in that moment of time, my brain is stressed."

I myself have witnessed his 'stressed' brain. His body quivers, standing is extremely difficult and he is washed with lethargy. When this happens David's brilliance is lost to sleep, but I see that in rest, his body is once again peaceful.

Before our session ends, David lets me know "in recent times, my world has shrunk". This is when I lean my head back and blink the tears away.

02:07

The time has come – when a 'lie' is not really a 'lie'

Mark Gibson

Mark Gibson manages an older people's mental health day services unit. This includes a day centre and outreach service for people suffering mental health issues, primarily dementia-type illnesses. The centre also works closely with other partners towards providing support and services to people with young onset diagnosis.

How many times must you correct your loved one? "I am not your sister, I am your wife." "I am not your father, I am your husband."

Then you try to explain – Mum died 15 years ago. You see the tears well up in your loved one's eyes. They did not know. No one told them. They start to grieve, again. This is the third time you have told them in as many days, and each time they grieve again. You feel the loss and hurt with them each time.

What do you do?

Lie. But to lie is not in your nature. You have always been taught not to lie. But surely to lie this time will avoid hurt, distress and trauma to your loved one.

"Mum is at work, she will be back later." You have done it. How did it feel? More importantly, how did your loved one react?

What I am saying is, is it really that bad that you told that white lie? After all it was to protect your loved one, and in truth it made that moment in time pass easier for yourself.

The hardest thing to come to terms with is that in some circumstances it is OK to tell that mistruth.

Now looking at that lie, mistruth, twist of actuality, what ever you want to call it – how bad is it when all you are doing is helping your loved one stay in that time in their mind, which is reality to them?

In my career in working among people with dementia I have had the most bizarre and surreal conversations with people, who believed it was still wartime, or the 1950s and so on. And in all those many conversations it was more calming for and accepted by the person with dementia for me to step into 'their world'.

'Their world', where Mum is next door. 'Their world', where Dad is asleep upstairs after his night shift. That is why we must be quiet. After all, he is never happy when we children wake him.

'Their world', the place where they truly believe they reside.

'Their world', where you, their mother, father, brother, sister, or whoever they believe you are at that time, can be happy and peaceful and content together.

Surely if that 'lie' helps, can it really be a 'lie'?

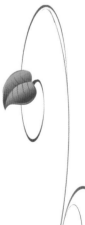
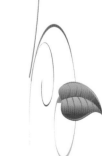

Slow flowing time

Richard Fleming

Richard Fleming is a clinical psychologist who has specialised in the development of services for people with dementia since the early 1980s. After working on the de-institutionalisation of elderly psychiatric hospital patients for the NSW Department of Health in Australia, he formed his own consultancy and then joined Hammond Care where, in 1996, he established the Dementia Services Development Centre. Richard and his staff have trained many thousands of aged care staff and contributed to the fields of environmental design and systematic care planning for people with dementia.

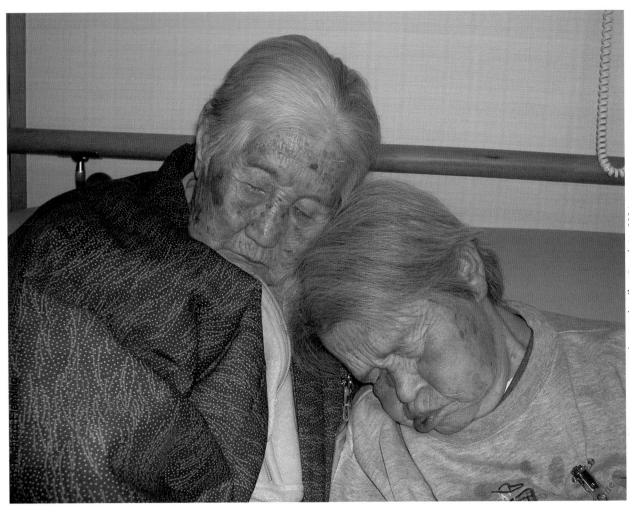

Sometimes opportunities arise to look at things from another point of view. A few years ago I was fortunate to be involved in writing a book (Fleming & Uchide 2004) that compared the care of people with dementia in a purpose designed Australian hostel with the care given in a Japanese group home. My Japanese co-author and I decided that the best way to explore the similarities and differences was to let the residents, staff and visitors take photographs of those things that they thought were essential to high quality care. So we gave them disposable cameras and the services of a professional photographer for three days in each place.

More than 1500 photographs were taken. Through a series of discussions with all concerned this collection was distilled to 30 photographs, 15 from each home.

In selecting the photographs we also tried to describe the themes they illustrated. The two interpreters we were working with were very skilled and sensitive. I remember two of their translations very clearly. Where I would have used the word 'observe' they translated the Japanese description as 'keeping a warm watch' and where I would have said 'spending time together' they interpreted the Japanese explanation as 'enjoying slow flowing time together'.

Spending time, coin by coin, second by second. As if it is ours to do what we like with, to spend it here or to spend it there.

But it isn't ours. It flows on whether we want to spend it or not and it has qualities of its own. Sometimes it is frenetically rapid, whirling us through the day gasping, and sometimes it flows slowly, supporting us while we enjoy being, perhaps alone, perhaps with others.

We are quite used to designing good traffic flows in environments for people with dementia. This usually involves making sure that the noisy, disruptive and unnecessary traffic is taken through an area that is separate from the living space. We know the benefits of allowing light to stream in (without making puddles of unknown depth on the floor). We arrange wandering paths so that they guide the movements of confused people, soothing their agitation by steering them to alternatives for their relentless pacing.

Maybe it is worth wondering about designing buildings that slow time down, that guide it into slow flowing eddies where we can enjoy time together?

Fleming R, Uchide Y (2004) *Images of Care in Australia and Japan: emerging common values.* Hammond Care Group & Tenjinkai Sonal Welfare Foundation, Sydney. Published by Dementia Services Development Centre, University of Stirling.

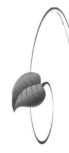

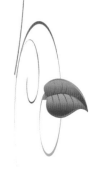

Time bends

Maria McManus

Maria McManus joined the Dementia Services Development Centre, University of Stirling in 2007. Maria is the Associate Director for the DSDC in Northern Ireland. She is an occupational therapist and has also completed an MBA in Health & Social Care and an MA, with distinction, in English (Creative Writing).

I am a clock; I am time,

measured in small pleasures;

I gaze into a gyre of lily pollen waltzing in Brownian motion where stone cups the rain –
it is the mirror of oceans;

or I am hunkered, launching leaf-boats; each helmed by a ladybird, navigating run-off under
hawthorn hedgerows.

These days, notions steer the hours, attracted into the nearness of little things and the fullness
of a single moment.

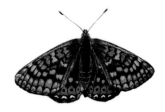

02:10

Time and time again

Malcolm Goldsmith

Malcolm Goldsmith is the author of *In A Strange Land, People with Dementia and the Local Church* and *Hearing the Voice of People with Dementia.* He worked for a while as a research fellow at the Dementia Services Development Centre in Stirling.

The ancient Greeks had two different words for time. *Kronos,* from which we get the world chronological, refers to time as an unwinding commodity. Twenty-four hours, 30 minutes, a year, a month or even a century. It is time which can be measured, arranged and planned. The other word is *Kairos,* which means something entirely different. Kairos means the appropriate moment or a significant fulfilment, when the 'time is right' or opportune. It relates to the content of the moment rather than the context. While kronos is quantitative, kairos is, by nature, qualitative.

There is little place for chronological time in the life of a person with dementia, but in the midst of ordinary time there is always the possibility of extraordinary time; there can always be a place for those transfiguring moments, those 'times' of contact, meaning and life-enhancing interaction. It does not matter what year the person with dementia appears to be living in, nor does it really matter what time of day or night it is (though I recognise that these can be real problems for carers). Chronological time is merely the movement of the spheres within the universe and we have calibrated this movement to give structure to our living. What matters for the person with dementia, no matter what 'time' they are living in, is this: is it possible to experience those feelings of well-being, those moments when their spirits are lifted and they become alive in a different way, when

they have that sense that "all shall be well and all manner of things shall be well"? Those are moments of transcendence, significant times breaking through the routine of chronological time.

For those of us who care for people with dementia, time can be a problem. We invariably have to live by diaries, clocks, meetings, appointments or routine. Time for medication, time for sleep, time for meals on a regular basis, time for the next doctor's appointment, we are driven by the '36 hour day' (Mace & Rabins 2006) This sort of time is essential for us if we are to live in the modern world and it can be extremely wearing. But for those people with dementia, what does it matter whether it is Friday or Tuesday, November or April, morning or afternoon? Time in that sense is meaningless. What does matter, and this is crucial, is that they are able to experience, grasp and enjoy those significant moments when they are at one with whatever time capsule they happen to be in at that moment, when they are at one with themselves and when those around them are able to allow, enable and appreciate the possibility of 'moments of meaning and significance'.

It is also important that those who care for people with dementia discover their own moments of transfiguration, when kairos can break through kronos in their own lives.

Mace N, Rabins P (2006) *The 36 Hour Day.* Johns Hopkins University Press, Baltimore.

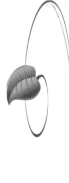
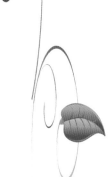

02:11

Cosmological time and dementia

Andrew Fairbairn

Andrew Fairbairn is a retired old age psychiatrist and was the Chair of the joint NICE/SCIE Guideline Development Group on Dementia.

My normal recreational reading is history, historical biography and politics. I suspect this is not unrelated to my clinical career of treating older people, because older people have both a history and their own memories of that lifetime.

I can never understand how some professionals could be interested in looking after children who, after all, have no history. Perhaps my children picked up this view when they were growing up!

In order to broaden my knowledge, I have been reading two or three 'amateur' paperbacks on cosmology, the space/time continuum, and a bit of quantum theory. I now feel a little bit more comfortable with how the basic particle theories break down when you get to a quantum level, and there was a moment when I understood how there could be seven dimensions instead of the conventional four, with three being in space and time. That moment did not last long, and it is completely beyond me how there could be a general consensus among quantum physicists that there are really eleven dimensions.

Oh, and incidentally, I don't understand 'red shift'. This is the idea, a bit like the Doppler effect in sound, that an expanding universe shifts light because the universe is expanding away from us as we look around us. However, we are on an obscure arm of a minor galaxy which is probably only one of billions, so how can there be universal expansion away from us when we are, by definition, not the centre of the universe?

As part of my struggling through these paperbacks, the concept of time becomes less and less clear. For example, I had thought that as matter was sucked in by the massive gravity of a black hole, one must cease to exist, but now I understand that it might just be an entry into another universe.

I had thought that standing on the edge of a black hole must involve some mass acceleration and an altered perception of time but, according to one article I read, there may be very little perception of change.

Increasingly, I am of the view that at a cosmological level, the concept of time is almost meaningless. Yet, to human beings, the concept of time is a vital, fundamental component of our everyday life as well as the key concept to the fact that we age. Losing a sense of time has always seemed frightening to me, but if the concept of time is so nebulous, maybe losing a sense of time is less awesome than I had originally imagined. Therefore, strangely, I wonder if there are parallels between a cosmological sense of time and dementia.

I feel confident that, notwithstanding the vast improvements in communication and information with people with dementia, there is still a point where insight into the disease process is lost. I had always imagined that this was a kind of perpetual purgatory. Of course the decline matters in terms of the dignity of the individual. It also matters for loved ones and other carers, as well as having an impact on society.

However, I am increasingly wondering if it does *not* matter to the person with dementia.

What day is it today?

Jane Gilliard

When I was young and newly married, long before I worked in dementia care, my father-in-law was diagnosed with Parkinson's disease. He coped well with his variable disability at first, but after my mother-in-law died he became very lonely and increasingly confused. He had several admissions to hospital and was assessed at different times. Eventually it was decided that he had dementia, probably vascular dementia, and he recognised that he needed more support. He moved into a nursing home near his former home in Lancashire. We lived at the other end of England in Somerset and visited him when we could.

Whenever we visited I noticed that he had a newspaper on the table next to his chair. The paper was always neatly folded, apparently unopened. I couldn't remember ever seeing my father-in-law reading a newspaper, so I wondered why he always had one in his room looking more like an ornament than something that was well thumbed and had been enjoyed. Maybe he was offered one by the staff at the nursing home as a way of his occupying himself. I was intrigued.

On one visit, my curiosity finally got the better of me. "Dad," I said to him, "I didn't realise you liked to read the paper." And his reply? "Oh, I don't read the paper. I buy it every day so that when the doctor comes to visit me and asks me what day it is today, I know I can give him the answer."

I couldn't help but wonder – how meaningful was it to ask this question of a man whose memory was sufficiently intact that he could remember that he would be asked and who had sufficient insight to take action to be sure he would know the answer!

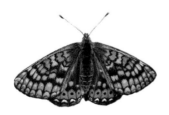

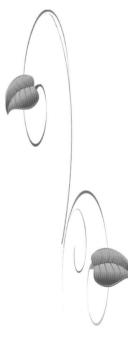

02:13

Too much time and not enough

John Holmes

John Holmes is a senior lecturer in liaison psychiatry of old age at the University of Leeds. He has clinical and research interests in novel approaches to mental health service delivery for older people, and in the management of co-morbid physical and mental health problems.

All night spent on the floor.
Time to feel the pain from the shards of bone in
  my hip.
Going to hospital in a blue-light rush.
Waiting in a cubicle where strangers come and go.
Fast-tracked to the ward in a four-hour hurry.

Time to be frightened in this strange place.
Time feeling thirsty with my drink out of reach but
  no time to find out how I like my tea.
Time feeling hungry.
Time to watch my food go cold.
No time to help me to eat.
Food taken away without time to eat.
Too much time on the bedpan.

Time to carry out tasks, but no time to talk to me.
Time to talk to the other patients but not to me.
Time to stand at the end of my bed talking about me
  not to me.
Time to spend chatting at the nursing station.
Time to talk with your colleagues about last night's TV.
Time to tick boxes but no time to care.

Time to feel the pain.
No time to give me painkillers.
Time to call for help.
No time to listen.
Time to tell me to shut up when I ask for help.
Time to tell me to sit down when I try to walk.
No time to find out what I want.

Time to give me drugs I don't need.
Time to put a needle in my arm but no time to tell
  me why.
Time to hear my children's wishes but not to
  hear mine.
Time to decide to move me to another strange place.
All too much time to forget the instructions from the
  physiotherapist.

Time to hurt.
Time to hope.
Time for hope to be dashed.
No time to try and get me back home where
  I belong.
A long time spent in hospital with no one to talk to.

I asked for help but no-one heard.
No one helped.
No one knew how.
Give me the time and help I need to recover.

Time to lose memories I'd rather not keep.

02:14

Indian Stretchable Time

Louise McCabe

Louise McCabe is a lecturer in dementia studies in the Dementia Services Development Centre at the University of Stirling. Louise's research and teaching interests focus on improving services and care practice for people with dementia in the UK and beyond.

In the UK we have GMT (Greenwich Mean Time) and BST (British Summer Time) and in India there is IST, Indian Standard Time or as my Indian friends call it, Indian Stretchable Time. Now means maybe later, this afternoon tomorrow and tomorrow probably at the start of next week.

As a Scottish PhD student undertaking research in Kerala, South India, I became acquainted with Indian Stretchable Time and both its frustration and its benefits. My research included observation and interviews and was undertaken in a day centre for people with dementia. For me at first IST was a barrier: I wanted to arrange times for interviews in advance but people were hard to pin down and when pinned down too far in advance (that is, anything more than a day) likely to be doing something else.

For my observations, though, IST was fine; I could sit and watch without any timetable or deadlines to meet. And what I observed was that IST works well for people with dementia. Here in the UK we are always stressing the need for flexibility and responsiveness within services for people with dementia. IST provides a simple solution – just do what needs doing now and let things fall into place.

At the day centre there was an order to things, first there was prayer, then reading the papers, then tea and so on. Each activity was given due attention and carried on until finished, then the next thing started. No rush to meet deadlines or achieve unnecessary goals – in fact I think we could all benefit from a bit of Stretchable Time.

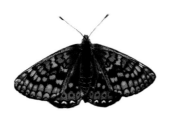

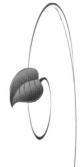

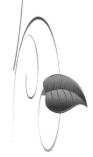

02:15

'And then there is Granny'

Trisha Kotai-Ewers

After years as a language teacher, Trisha Kotai-Ewers began working as a writer with people with dementia in 1997, following the example of John Killick in the UK. Her book on the words of people with dementia, *Listen to the Talk of Us: People with dementia speak out*, was published by Alzheimer's Australia (WA) in 2007.

It wasn't as if Jane spoke about time. The word does not appear in my notes of her conversations. She simply lived time in a different way to the rest of us. Let me try to explain.

When I met her, Jane lived in a dementia-specific hostel. And yet, her words told me that she lived on the family farm of her childhood. Everyone who shared her space at the hostel was identified as someone on the farm, as she pointed them out to me. An ageing nun was 'Mary-Ann', who she assured me was not a relative. As another woman resident approached the dining table Jane announced: "And there's Granny."

Women staff members wearing slacks became the men on the farm. "They're good boys... they know how to look after things." That transposition fascinated me. In part it reflected Jane's origins in an era when only men wore trousers. But her words revealed the metaphor underlying the obvious parallel between the clothes worn by hostel staff and the men on her childhood farm. Staff members were as much in control within the hostel world as those men had been. They all knew "how to look after things".

In some respects this 'past in the present' element in Jane's conversation felt like a natural expression of the importance her past life had assumed. But on our second meeting her words shook me out of any complacency. Noticing that one man's name recurred frequently in her narrative I asked if he was her husband. "Not yet!" she replied with a twinkle in her eye. While living her past within the framework of her present, Jane retained an awareness of future events, or rather, of events which from the vantage point of the distant past still belonged to her future. From the point of the present, the event definitely lay in the past. I can feel my mind wobbling on its axis of accepted knowledge even as I attempt to describe this.

It felt as if Jane viewed her daily life through different frames, each one transparent, so that past, present and future could all be seen at the same time, while still retaining their own identity and reality. Perhaps she was simply expressing that complex teaching of both ancient metaphysics and today's quantum physics – that past, present and future, rather than being in strict linear procession, are in fact all happening at the same moment.

How can we, as carers, deal with such transparency of time in the experience of the people with dementia for whom we care? How can we find a point of balance between the demands time places on our lives and the apparent timelessness in which some people with dementia seem to live. We need to become a little less firmly anchored in society's determination to keep past, present and future in neatly sequestered boxes that follow one after the other. Perhaps we can then find space to enter acceptingly into the world as they see it. In the process, perhaps we can learn to move a little more fluidly from present to past to the future which exists within the past. Perhaps, learning this, we might escape the tyranny with which clock time regulates our days and our need to be constantly 'doing'. And in that space and fluidity, perhaps we might come to dwell more on 'being' and so learn possibly the greatest lesson people with dementia can teach us: it is who we are that matters far more than what we do.

02:16

Time

Jean Tottie

Jean Tottie is an occupational therapist. She was seconded for two years to the Northern & Yorkshire Regional Office of the NHS Executive to manage implementation of the National Service Framework for Older People; helped to set up the first Dementia Services Collaborative; worked in a primary care trust on redesign of older people's services; and was Network Director for Older People's Services across Greater Manchester. She took early retirement when her father needed more care and support as his dementia advanced. Jean now works voluntarily to improve services for people with dementia and specifically for the charity *for dementia*. She was a carer on one of the external reference groups developing the National Dementia Strategy.

Hi Dad. Have you had a good day? Hasn't it been lovely today? "Oh yes, I've been busy as usual."

Did you manage to get out in the garden, then?

"No, I didn't have enough time."

Oh, what have you been up to then? Painting?

"No, I had too much to do around the house."

That's good. We can do some gardening together tomorrow if it stays fine.

This was a typical conversation I had with Dad when I phoned him each day whilst he was living alone at home, with dementia. Dad could still recall that he used to have a routine of household chores and assumed that he still did them. In reality, I had been doing his cleaning and laundry for some time but he still loved his garden and would potter about in his shed or greenhouse for hours.

As a keen watercolourist, always with a painting on the go, he would say he didn't have enough time to get on with it and yet he didn't know what he had been doing all day. As Dad's dementia progressed, his daily routine slipped such that he needed regular prompts by his home care assistant and me to look at the clock. He was often up before dawn and going for his morning walk round the local country park in the dark in all weathers.

Did you see the ladies with their dogs this morning Dad?

"No, I didn't today."

When asked what time he went out for his walk – "the usual time". Dad had no concept of time in his routine by now. He would have his meals earlier and earlier, then go to bed early and get up early!

Dad wasn't worried or anxious. He had no insight into his dementia, but he was getting socially isolated.

Soon after this, following a short spell in hospital due to an infection, Dad went to live in a residential home where he made new friends. He didn't have any chores to do and so had plenty of time to mix with other people and go for walks. After all, his daily routine was now managed by the care staff so he didn't have to worry about getting his jobs done.

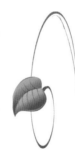
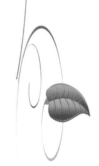

02:17

Reflections past and present

Suzanne Cahill

Dr Suzanne Cahill is a Research Senior Lecturer and Director of the research programme of DSIDC (The Dementia Services Information and Development Centre) within St James Hospital Dublin and School of Social Work and Social Policy, Trinity College, Dublin.

Recently I stayed in a friend's thatched cottage in the West of Ireland. The area, known locally as 'Eannach Mhian', is in the Gaeltacht (all Irish-speaking locale) and is connected to the mainland by bridge.

Once a day, a bus from Galway stops at the local garage or wherever you choose to dismount. The local people are primarily engaged in farming, fishing and tourism. They live a simple but one would suspect peaceful life. Here, little houses can be seen speckled across the landscape, man-made walls, relics of old stone cottages never demolished, Celtic emblems, a church with its adjoining cemetery. Brightly painted anchored fishing boats can be heard lapping against the shores as the large over-fed sheepdog saunters up the road. Even the cattle and sheep seem to stroll languidly around the roads and time is of no real consequence. It is a magnificently remote tranquil scene, so isolated that when I asked a local shop-keeper where a certain boreen (Irish word for little dirt road) led to, he took endless time to draw me a map and then, in passing, reminded me that the next stop was America!

So, you may well ask yourself, what is the connection between this idyllic holiday spot and the topic of time and dementia? Interestingly, the West and North West of Ireland have the largest proportion of older people in Eire and consequently the highest percentage of people diagnosed with Alzheimer's disease. Yet what struck me as strange was that during the entire sojourn there, we never once encountered an elderly man or woman with an obvious cognitive impairment, nor did I see even one nursing home or retirement village, despite the multiple signposts for B & Bs and hair salons throughout the countryside.

This has left me wondering where older frail and disabled people in the West now live? What happens when they become highly dependent or develop a dementia and need long-term care? Are they relocated to cities or are rural nursing homes situated in even more isolated areas where our elderly people are 'socially marooned', further distanced from all they once knew and loved? Ireland, like other countries, now has an influx of migrant workers, mainly Polish, Latvian and Lithuanian, many of whom work as paid caregivers. How do migrant staff communicate with people with dementia from this part of Ireland whose only language is Gaielge (Irish Gaelic)? Are they given extra time in their caregiving duties given the complexities involved?

Fast forward to Dublin, where I am working on a research study on quality of life and dementia in long-stay care. At the first nursing home I visited, I am particularly struck by two very harsh notices on display in the facility's porch:

(i) To comply with HSE regulations, all visitors must wash their hands before entrance

(ii) To comply with fire regulations, all visitors must sign in and out of the visitors book.

My mind reflects back to the West, to the traditional Irish cottages, with their hall doors wide open during the long hot summer days, and the sheepdog barking at the back of the old hay barn. The contrast is stark and disturbing. How might those whose earlier lives were spent in such idyllic settings now feel being enclosed in such clinical and austere environments?

I ring the doorbell at this nursing home and after a long pause, a clatter of keys can be heard jangling from outside. It is as if Fort Knox is being opened. On entry, several residents are sitting near the main door. One has her crossword in hand. She tells me she is 96 and is very proud of the fact that she does the crossword every day. Today she is doing the more complicated one. Another potters up the corridor and proceeds to interview me in a rather charming way as I wait to be told where I am going. Like many nursing homes, the entrance hall is the hub where many residents congregate.

The study which has brought me here, entails doing MMSEs (Mini Mental State Examinations) and MOCAs (Montreal Cognitive Assessments) on residents, some of whom have a dementia. I begin by asking them to talk about life in this nursing home. What is important now, what brings joy and sadness to their lives? Overwhelmingly most seem remarkably content with life and appear genuinely satisfied with the care received. They love having visitors, the outings arranged by the nursing home and the activity programme. These people have much in common – they want to talk and be listened to, and they all have plenty of time. Discussions then lead me to doing the tests. The schedule is to complete five interviews a day and I am conscious of time constraints having assured staff I will be in and out in no time.

However, administering these tests means asking many questions, a much less pleasant experience for all, since these are people who wish to talk spontaneously and not be interrogated. They are people who need time to talk and to think – a dimension clearly not factored into these respective scales. Some are profoundly deaf and have huge difficulty hearing the actual questions. Several have chronic disabilities due to arthritis or Parkinson's disease for example, or following a stroke, and consequently are unable to undertake certain aspects of the test such as paper-folding, sentence-writing and copy-drawing. Many are clearly aware of their deficits and seem embarrassed at having them exposed.

And now, a week later, writing up these experiences, I have time to ponder and reflect. How and why should one be expected to know the day, if each day in this nursing home is essentially the same as the next? And is knowing what season it is really relevant if you are wheelchair bound, have no next of kin and have not been taken outdoors for some two years? And if you are 97 and tell a stranger that you live in St Margaret's when the nursing home is now called St Catherine's (although formerly St Margaret's) does this really warrant a score of 0? And finally, is it fair and ethical to bombard these vulnerable people with such probing questions – many of which are totally irrelevant to their current lives?

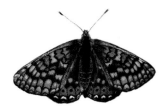

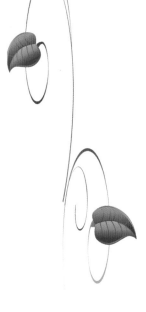

02:18

Ahead of his time

Charlotte Clarke

Charlotte Clarke is Professor of Nursing Practice Development Research and Associate Dean for Research in the School of Health, Community and Education Studies at Northumbria University. Charlotte worked clinically with older people for several years and now focuses on undertaking a variety of research activities which aim to develop healthcare practices.

1980s
Rehabilitation ward they called it
But few ever left alive

Edward
Let's call him that
Wordlessly seeing out his days
Silent with his fragile dignity

Early shift
Time to get Edward up
Talking – monologue
Not expecting any answer

Gardening
Edward's job in years before
Lettuce and the problem of slugs

Slug pellets, salt rings, jars of beer
Tried them all
Any suggestions?

"Don't grow them"
A silence broken!
But instantly returns
Forever, for Edward

I don't grow lettuce now
Such ecological wisdom
Didn't think like that in the 80s
So ahead of his time

Few words, big lesson
That has shaped my life
Work with, not against
Thank you Edward.

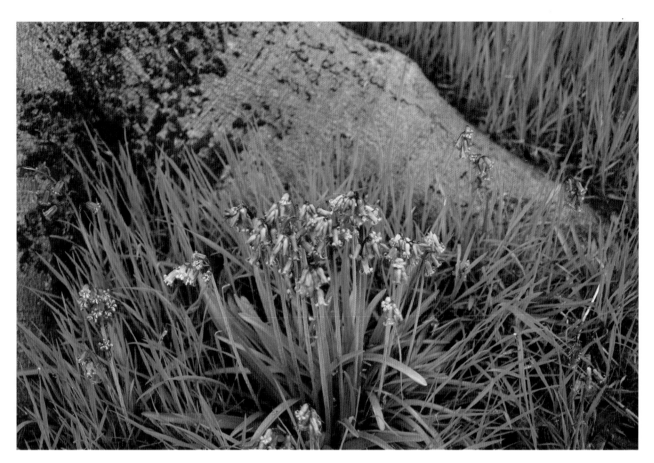

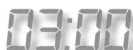

Making time

03:01

Dementia time, doctor time

David & Susan Jolley

David Jolley MSc FRCPsych. pioneered services for older people in the North West of England from 1975, and was Professor of Old Age Psychiatry and Medical Director in Wolverhampton 1995-2003. He maintains part-time activities: clinical for Tameside and Glossop, and academic at the Personal Social Services Research Unit, Manchester University and Dementia Services Development Centre, West Midlands.

Susan Jolley MB ChB MRCPsych. was a Consultant Old Age Psychiatrist in South Manchester from 1982-1985.

Albert Kushlick (Blunden & Kushlick 1975) called us (the doctors) 'hit and run' merchants – in for a quick assessment, perhaps a letter and a domiciliary claim, and on to the next scenario. In this he contrasted our contribution and depth of knowledge and understanding with the eight hour shift of nurses and professional carers and the 24 hours a day every day of family (Barker 1999). The notion was extended to the 36-hour day by Nancy Mace and Peter Rabins (Mace & Rabins 2006)

Kushlick was perceptive and right of course. He was drawing attention to the power and responsibilities of doctors to influence care, treatment, the provision of resource and the relatively fragile baseline from which they (are content to) work, and for which they are very well paid.

In contrast, those who really know are little valued and lack influence.

But doctors can and do stick around. Some have given 30 years and more professional commitment to dementia as a concept and to generations of individuals and families with the condition. This carries the opportunity and responsibility to see people through: being there for individuals, families and colleagues throughout the course of months and years of changing strengths, weaknesses and needs, to an end that is sometimes awful. Tom Arie emphasised this as one of the key attributes of a successful psychogeriatric service (Arie 1981). We hope that this is still honoured.

In addition there is the broader responsibility to hold true to what we know of basic and essential principles of good care, through advances in knowledge, possibilities of new treatments and serial well-intentioned, political and policy-driven changes in the infrastructure of 'welfare'. Being there, being unashamed and carrying, as banners to be proud of, the stigmas associated with age, impairment and loss of legal competence which cling to dementia by whatever name.

It is so easy to be diverted by directives from above or the flatteries or criticisms of colleagues.

Arie T (1981) *Health Care of the Elderly.* Croom Helm.
Barker P (1999) *The philosophy and practice of psychiatric nursing.* Churchill Livingstone, Edinburgh.
Blunden R, Kushlick A (1975) Looking for practical solutions. *Age Concern Today* 13: 2-5.
Mace N, Rabins, P (2006) *The 36 hour day.* Johns Hopkins University Press, Baltimore.

03:02

A game of frustration

Anon

If you insist or push me a lot
the very thing you want to happen – will not
The opposite will occur
you'll confuse and unnerve me
I will stutter and slur

If I'm lucky I'll be able to locate the word
it doesn't match or fit, it's not the one I want heard
it has no relevancy
I'm losing all fluency

Words blur, I mix up vowels and consonants
I lose all sense in the sentence
Please don't demand, let me be
only then will I trust you not to humiliate me
don't challenge or hurry me, I'll become mute
only time and patience will bear fruit

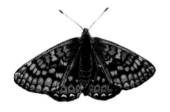

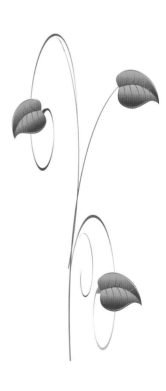

03:03

Daily life in care homes: minute by minute

Penny Banks & Rhidian Hughes

Penny Banks was Head of Information and Reporting at the Commission for Social Care Inspection, responsible for the publication of CSCI special studies and reports, including the annual report to Parliament on the state of social care in England. Penny previously worked at the King's Fund where she led a national programme on support to carers and had a number of studies on policy and practice in social care published, including some on the care market and integrated care for older people. Penny is currently a member of the Standing Commission on Carers.

Dr Rhidian Hughes worked for the Commission for Social Care Inspection and was responsible for a number of studies including *See me, not just the dementia*, which examined the quality of care for people with dementia in care homes. He now works for the Care Quality Commission. He also holds honorary positions as a visiting senior lecturer at Guy's, King's and St Thomas' School of Medicine and a visiting senior research fellow at the Institute of Gerontology, King's College London.

How people spend time during the day in care homes is crucial to their quality of life. Even more so for people with dementia who may find it difficult to care for themselves and communicate with those around them. These problems bring care homes considerable challenges to ensure staff understand and communicate well with people with dementia. So too, there are challenges for regulators seeking to judge service quality through people's direct experiences. The Care Quality Commission, which replaced the former social care regulator for England, the Commission for Social Care Inspection (CSCI) in 2009, is seeking ways to understand people's experiences of care better, minute by minute.

Assessing the quality of care

People want to maintain their privacy and dignity and have choice and control about their care. CSCI introduced a new observational approach to help inspectors get closer to the perspectives and experiences of people so that better judgements can be made about service quality.

The Short Observational Framework for Inspection (Brooker *et al*, 2007) builds on Dementia Care Mapping (Brooker 2005), a powerful approach towards understanding the quality of care people receive from the perspective of the individual. Inspections using the Short Observational Framework

for Inspection (SOFI) involve two hours of continuous observation of five people. Every five minutes inspectors make recordings, looking in detail at individuals' emotional well-being, what they are doing, with whom, and how staff relate to them.

These five-minute units of analysis illustrate some interesting patterns in the ways in which people with dementia spend their time in care homes. In the very best situations, SOFI can reveal care that provides maximum dignity and respect to individuals.

See me, not just the dementia

CSCI's report *See me, not just the dementia* is the first in-depth observational study, of 424 people with dementia living in 100 care homes (CSCI 2008). About 840 hours of people's experiences were analysed. During busy times of day when observations took place (eg mealtimes), we found people were occupied, either alone or with someone else, during 73% of their time. However, we also identified 57 people (13%) who spent less then 30 minutes of their time engaged with the world around them and some people were withdrawn. People who were less active tended to be those individuals with the most severe communication problems.

Communication has a tremendous impact on how people feel. Negative, disrespectful or frank questions or commands lower people's moods. But friendly and warm exchanges leave people feeling happy and relaxed. One inspector illustrates this point in his report:

"One carer was observed throughout the entire inspection to interact positively with residents, providing warmth, acknowledgement and respect of individuals' needs. Several residents were observed to respond to this carer by either smiling, providing good eye contact or by making positive verbal comments. When questioned by the inspector the carer was clearly knowledgeable of individual residents' care needs, personal preferences, likes and dislikes. One resident was overheard to say as the carer left the lounge area 'she's lovely' and 'I like her'." (Inspection Report)

This quotation illustrates some of the key elements of good practice where staff fully understand each individual and take time to get to know them, their needs and wishes. Another inspector comments positively on how one care home encouraged people to establish and maintain their routines:

"One person has got an ironing board in her bedroom so she can do her own ironing. It was observed during the inspection that people living in the home were able to follow their own routine, getting up more slowly if they wished to do so and spending time in their bedrooms if they preferred. Two of the residents said they liked to stay up later and watch TV in the lounge." (Inspection Report)

Supporting positive practice

The CSCI study compared the characteristics of the top band of homes performing well in communicating with people with those in the lowest band. There was little difference between those homes performing well and those performing poorly in terms of the built environment and whether the home specialised in the care of people with dementia. Instead the key ingredients that support positive practice are:

- A care home ethos that puts people first and promotes their dignity and respect at all times
- Strong leadership and senior staff who provide a role model in good communication and care
- Good support for staff and working conditions that encourage people to stay in their job, as well as high quality training and development opportunities.

Conclusion

There are nearly a quarter of a million people with dementia living in care homes, and the figures are projected to rise considerably over the next few years. The quality of care is vitally important for people in their final years and months of life. Examining how people spend their time, minute by minute, allows the regulator to get beyond the surface of routine adequate care practice to reveal care that provides maximum dignity and respect to individuals and, most importantly, to drive improvements in the quality of care for people with dementia.

Brooker D (2005) Dementia Care Mapping (DCM): a review of the research literature. *Gerontologist* 45 11-18.

Brooker D, May H, Walton S *et al* (2007) Introducing SOFI: a new tool for inspection of care homes. *Journal of Dementia Care* 15(4) 22-24.

Commission for Social Care Inspection (CSCI) (2008) *See me, not just the dementia. Understanding people's experiences of living in a care home.* Commission for Social Care Inspection, London. A full report and interactive CD-ROM version with filmed interviews is available on the report is available on the Care Quality Commission website: http://www.cqc.org.uk/_db/_documents/Dementia%20Report-web.pdf

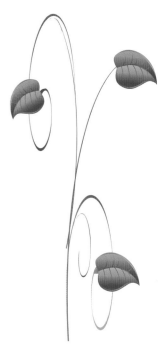

03:04

The dictator time

Sally Knocker

Sally Knocker is part-time Director of Communications for NAPA, the National Association for Providers of Activities for Older People, and a freelance trainer and writer in dementia care. Sally trained as a drama therapist and is involved in intergenerational arts projects in care homes with the charity Magic Me and as a trustee of the theatre company Ladder to the Moon.

"When you have finished your jobs, please try and find time to talk to the residents."

This was a notice seen on a wall in a care home, written by a presumably desperate manager. This prompted me to write the following. It is not intended as a dig at care home staff, many of whom frequently tell me on training days how frustrating they find the constraints on their time and the pressure to conform to established routines. Managers also tell me that they don't want their staff to be so controlled by the rigidity of time. Yet the voice below is still out there somewhere, and if it is not from the manager or the care workers, whose is the voice and where is it coming from?

Got to get everyone up for breakfast on time.

Beds need to be made by 10am!

Standards to be maintained!

Time to take a stroll round the block with someone who likes to walk?

Maybe later.

Care plans to be done, rotas to be organised, email mountains to climb.

The inspectors are coming!

Stars in our eyes!

Lunch must be served at 12.30 pm

Even though people are having fun in the garden with a visiting dog.

Sorry, no time for that!

Tick Tock.

Come now, no time to dawdle!

The kitchen staff need to clear up before shifts end.

No time to talk – there is REAL work to be done!

Fancy a cuppa at 2.30? 'No dear, the trolley is coming at 3.'

Tea is at 3pm - On the DOT.

Tick, Tock.

2-3pm – we DO the activities. That's when the staff has a bit of time.

Time on your own? Not really, we want everyone to have a jolly time!

Knees up Mother Brown.

Tick, Tock.

Must get everyone to bed on time or the night staff will grumble!

Tick, Tock

NO TIME TO

STOP.

Please let us unwrap time from the tyranny of the institutional CLOCK and allow it to be S p o n t a n e o u s And Precious - For *people* Again.

03:05

'I haven't got time' – truth or untruth?

Chris Sherratt

Chris Sherratt has been involved in dementia care as professional, volunteer and carer for a number of years, and now works for Dementia Care Consulting in Bristol, England (www.dementiacareconsulting.co.uk). His contribution reflects his concern about the gap between aspirations and reality in many areas of dementia care.

"**I**'m sorry, I can't help you, I haven't got time." We use the excuse a lot, and it can't always be true. Here is a scenario:

In a care home, a resident sitting in the lounge (call him Jack) calls out to a care worker (Kath) who is passing the door: "Nurse, I want to go to the toilet." Kath calls out "I haven't got time, Jack", or "I'll be with you in a minute", and continues on her way.

This could be absolutely true. Maybe another wing of the home is on fire and Kath has to help to evacuate the residents! Or it could be absolutely untrue, if Kath is desperate for a smoke, and gives any excuse. But in between these two unlikely absolutes, 'I haven't got time' could still be a truthful answer – or not. It all depends.

Let us assume that Kath, like most care workers, is busy, with a number of things to do, and she very probably knows that even if she gets them all done she hasn't got time to do them all as well as she would like. When she tells Jack that she 'hasn't got time', she is going through two processes. First let us assume that if Jack were on the floor, Kath would stop whatever she was doing at the time and go to help him. Likewise, she would probably also respond immediately if she knew that Jack never normally asked for help, as it would suggest that he was facing something of an emergency. So Kath has made a quick assessment that there is no

emergency requiring her immediate attention. She also decides that the things she is already doing are more important than taking Jack to the toilet at that moment, so she is prioritising the things she needs to do. She may come back later, or ask someone else to help Jack, but this is part of her prioritising.

So far it is perhaps a part-truth for Kath to say "I haven't got time". Suppose however that Kath knows that Jack was taken to the toilet 10 minutes ago. Maybe Kath took him herself, and maybe she knows that even if she stops to remind Jack he will not remember, and will still insist, as this happens every day. In this case Kath assesses that Jack is asking for something that he does not need, and prioritises that this is not as important as the number of other things she has to do at the moment. A truthful answer would be "But you went to the toilet 10 minutes ago", but Kath knows that this will not solve the problem, so she says "I haven't got time".

But suppose that Jack calls out frequently. He is labelled an 'attention-seeker'. His care plan might even say (as some do) that staff should not respond when Jack calls out, as this only encourages him to call out more. It is easier for Kath to say "I haven't got time" than to say "Sorry Jack... you're only calling for attention" or even "I'm not allowed to come and talk to you". But in this example it

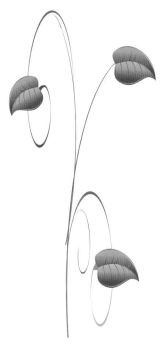

is clear that when Kath says "I haven't got time", she is not telling the truth.

As these examples progress, Kath begins to appear something of a villain, with increasing levels of dishonesty. But let's not blame Kath. She would say that she is 'only doing her best', and that her response to Jack was a kindly way of avoiding becoming involved when she had more important things to do.

Here we have to ask what things are more important than helping Jack to go to the toilet? Suppose that Kath has promised another resident that she will take them to the toilet, and then help them to get dressed, and then…? Fair enough, but a bit of positive negotiation between the residents would be more considerate to both of them than leaving Jack unattended. It is common for care staff to feel that they have too much to do, and therefore nearly inevitable that some assessment and prioritising will be necessary. So apart from the obvious conclusion that more staff hours are needed ('hours' are not the same as 'time'), it is important to train staff in the use of their time, and how they manage these processes of assessing and prioritising – minute events in themselves, but so important.

Frequently, at the moment when Jack (and the thousands of people that Jack represents in this example) calls out to Kath, he does not really need to go to the toilet. What he wants, perhaps needs, is some attention, some time to be given to him, and it is this kind of time that Kath does not have. The Alzheimer's Society report *Home from Home* (2007) tells us that some residents can spend only two minutes in six hours interacting with staff or other residents. Jack probably only gets his two minutes, but he is too restless to allow himself to become bored by doing nothing, and his ability to initiate some activity himself is impaired. So he calls for attention in the only way that he can think of.

This does not need to be the case. When someone does take Jack to the toilet, or even, let us say, when a person with profound disabilities is given a bed bath, these practical tasks need to take place in a setting of social interaction, where the person comes first, rather than the task to be done. This will increase significantly the amount of time that residents spend interacting with other people, and is the key to giving real time, quality time to people with dementia in any care setting.

This does mean providing more staff hours, but the real way to create time is for managers to move their own priorities away from physical care (what we used to call 'feeding and watering') and to give their staff the space (this means time) and the skills to develop value-based communication with residents. When Jack called to Kath, she didn't tell the truth, but sadly it was the only way she knew how to respond.

Alzheimer's Society (2007) *Home from home.*

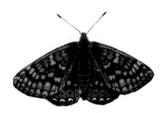

03:06

Time present

Tony Price

Tony Price has been writing and directing programmes for some 25 years. Before that he was a film editor, which requires patience. More recent programmes through the Cast Iron Film Company have focused on mental health issues where patience is again essential. Shots and sequences have to develop on their own – things cannot be forced to happen to a schedule. The results are programmes that explain subjects such as dementia with clarity and understanding.

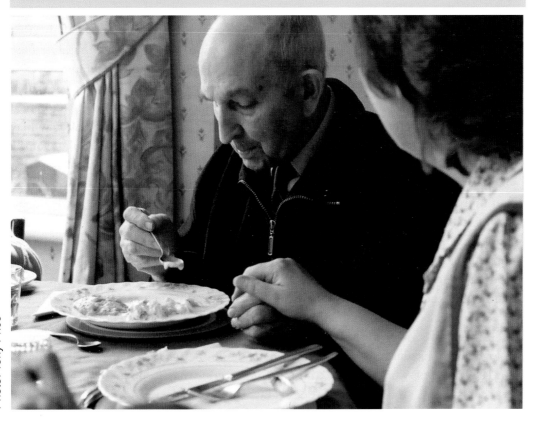

Photo: Tony Price

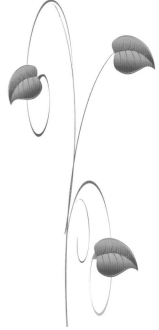

We all do things at different speeds. This is never more true than with eating. At this care home staff eat their meals alongside the residents and not surprisingly the staff tend to finish their meals earlier. Yet they remain at the table to encourage and help so that an air of calm pervades the dining room. In this frame the resident doesn't need help to eat, but by holding his hand the member of staff is reassuring him that there is no hurry. He can take his time. Clearing away and the clattering of plates can happen later.

03:07

The privilege of caring

Deborah Sturdy

Deborah Sturdy is Nurse Advisor for Older People at the Department of Health, London. She has been working in the field of older people nursing for most of her career as a researcher, clinician, manager and most recently at a national level in policy development. She has worked across primary, acute, independent and social care settings. Her most rewarding clinical post was working with people with dementia in Bristol.

One of the many challenges of nursing is delivering individual care. It is not about the understanding of its meaning, rather that it proves to be such a huge challenge in its application to practice. The guilt and the tension experienced in trying to do the right thing at the right time for patients is mentally exhausting as the external forces and demands of multiple tasks take hold on the limitations of time.

My career since qualifying as a nurse has thrown up many challenges but time is the constant battle. First in to work on the early shift and last out at night has been a life-long habit. Even giving beyond the expectations of my contract never seemed to suffice – and that was without taking home the guilt of what I'd not done rather than what I had achieved in my working day.

When I reflect on the 23 years of a rich career, the one job I would return to tomorrow is senior sister on a dementia ward. The challenges of working with people with complex health needs and with an underlying dementia in an acute hospital was the best job I have had. The challenges of the clinical environment and complexity of care provided me with the exact mixture which had attracted and inspired me to be a nurse. It was where 'nursing' came into its own, working in such a challenging environment.

Eighteen patients, all with complex needs; a staffing complement, which was insufficient; and an environment, which was the back ward of the 'workhouse' – this was not so inspirational. How could you realistically care for so many people providing individual care and therapy? Honestly? With great difficulty. The compromise was using that little time you had for any one person to the maximum effect. It was getting to know the person as best you could within the environment in which you were and, most importantly, being flexible. What worked today may not work tomorrow when getting co-operation for the simplest of tasks. Why have a battle about an approach if it's not going to work? It would take twice as long for no outcome other than frustration.

Using time effectively for me was about talking, laughing, tuning in to a level of understanding and compromise. Adapting every day to the little time you had for that one person and making that time work for both of you. Investing in knowing that person was the best investment of all. The chocolate bribe for one person getting dressed, or singing a song with another made life better for us all. The routine of hospital life certainly has its limitations. However, it doesn't take much to make it work for you rather than against you. Taking someone for a walk with me when I had to go to the pharmacy or hospital office provided both therapy and snatched moments for that person. One to one we could have a different dialogue, a purposeful 'wander' along the corridors or through the gardens, minutes longer to my task in hand but to stop and smell the roses and feel the sun were benefits that were priceless. It is about being flexible with time when caring, but most importantly it's about using your imagination.

03:08

Taking time to save time

David Gribble

David Gribble works for Alzheimer's Australia WA. His job encompasses strategic project management and service development for the organisation, and he is currently overseeing its new focus on research and development, dementia risk reduction and healthy ageing strategies. David is currently undertaking PhD studies at Curtin University Graduate School of Business, researching aspects of the aged care sector in Australia.

Talking to care staff about how to interact more effectively with people with dementia is a common aspect of dementia care education. Good communication is central to good dementia care, and it hinges on getting to know the person; their life, loves, needs, motivations and desires. Knowing the person with dementia means we can establish a connection with them more easily and may be able to anticipate their needs before they manifest themselves as behaviours that we may find 'challenging'.

When we talk about this need to learn about the person, one of the commonest things we hear careworkers say is, "But I don't have the time! How can I find out what makes the person 'tick' when I have to provide care for them and there aren't enough hours in the day?"

A good question, and one that is increasingly relevant for aged care as it struggles with staff shortages and demands for efficiency and cost-effectiveness. The answer, of course, lies in the need to be empowered to take a slightly longer-term view of our interactions with the person than just the immediate care task required. Just as politicians often have difficulty planning beyond the next election, we can also struggle with the idea of doing some initial investiga-tion and planning in order to make a future task easier.

If we can take a longer view, we see that we are likely to be providing the same care task repeatedly over a fairly long period of time. If this task is more difficult because it is not meeting the needs of the person with dementia and they are not a willing participant, then we need to think about all the extra time that the activity is adding up to for us and them. If instead we have taken the time to learn about the person, know what their needs are and plan accordingly, then the task may well take less time with their active involvement, thus saving us significant time (and stress) over the longer term.

Multiply one care task or activity that is achieved more quickly through communica-tion and planning by the thousands of interactions we have each week and we can start to see that a little bit of forethought and understanding can make a considerable difference – not only to the time we have available to care, but also to the quality of our interactions and relationships with people with dementia.

And better relationships means a less stressed carer and a more content person with dementia – and that is surely worth the time…

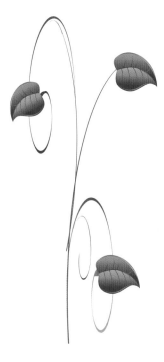

03:09

No time to hang around!

Gwyn Grout

Gwyn Grout works within the NHS as a Consultant Nurse. As part of her role she provides, develops and evaluates services for older people with mental health problems who find themselves in hospital. This also involves enabling general hospital staff to develop their knowledge and skills.

The focus of my clinical and research attention is caring for older people with mental health problems in the general hospital setting. The concept of time, or lack of it, is frequently cited as the reason for challenges in meeting the needs of people with dementia appropriately while they are in hospital.

To illustrate these perceptions I draw on information from my research that examined how mental health problems in old age are perceived in the hospital setting (Grout 2007). I interviewed a total of 58 older people, relatives and staff members. The names that I use are not the real names of the people I interviewed.

The perception of mental health problems in old age in the general hospital setting is (broadly speaking) of a group of people who do not fit in with normal hospital business, and therefore take up too much time that should properly be directed towards medical issues. Arnold, an older man in hospital, went as far as saying that a mental health problem in old age is defined by "the time consumed by nursing staff". These people, he asserted, take up a disproportionate amount of time. And "they [the staff] don't have the time to care for that sort of person".

Some of the respondents linked the inability of staff to give time to an apparent stigma, an avoidance of accepting that the care of older people with mental health problems forms part of a professional's role in this setting. George, a man who had dysphasia and some memory changes said that "the staff do not give you time when you have had a stroke and can't think so well as you used to". He went on to describe how he has not been afforded the time to consider issues about how, and where, his future care needs would be met. Malcolm suggests that his wife was not given a drink because the staff did not feel that somebody with her condition (Alzheimer's disease) warranted their time.

"They didn't have time to hold a cup of liquid to her mouth." Pat, whose mother has memory problems, but "not that bad", describes "the noisy people are taking [the nurses'] time away. As Louisa, an older patient, says, "[the staff] haven't got time to just hang around".

Even those staff who work within the speciality of caring for older people, and demonstrate considerable skill in recognising and meeting the needs of people with cognitive problems, were critical of the extra time required, time that potentially could be spent doing their 'proper' jobs. Nurse Christine resents the fact that older people with mental health problems are transferred to her ward because others, in acute medical wards, do not have time or the patience to work with them: "The main problem we have is the very wandery patients who take up a huge chunk of your time." Dr Diane confirms: "They all take so much time. They just need someone to sit with them." Nurse Trish reiterates the point in saying that "it is very difficult for us when we are nursing people who are medically ill. We don't have time to sit with them and explain that they are safe and that their relatives know where they are". Daughter Helen sums up the majority view that "if the nurses have to look after mentally ill people they don't have time for their proper jobs", taking blood pressure etc.

Few of the interviewees considered that the older people with mental health problems, who they perceive as using too much time, have the right to be in an acute hospital. Notably this research was carried out in 2005/6. It is pleasing to report that focus on general hospital care for people with dementia is already challenging and changing the perceptions described above.

Grout G (2007) *Now you see them, Now you don't: Mental Health Problems in old age in the General Hospital setting.* University of Surrey (unpublished PhD).

03:10

The clock is ticking

Alan Chapman

Before his recent retirement Alan Chapman was Associate Director (Education and Training) at the Dementia Services Development Centre, University of Stirling in Scotland, and tutor/co writer of the post-graduate MSc in Dementia Studies module: Education and Support for Dementia Care Workers.

It is an alarming experience for any trainer to arrive at a venue to discover that the equipment requested has not been provided, the room is cold and chairs are not set out. The clock ticks towards the start time for the course. In a mild panic the trainer rushes about getting things sorted. Some participants then arrive 40 minutes early because their manager told them the wrong start time. Still no coffee or tea. They become silent onlookers as the increasingly frantic trainer finds that the overhead projector cable and laptop need an extension lead, and the flip-chart stand is broken. Other participants arrive and restlessness sets in as there are grumbles about having to wait for coffee/tea. The clock ticks – it is the start of the course and the trainer decides to start with a group exercise – to buy time!

Although perhaps an exaggeration of what can go wrong the above scenario is familiar to many trainers. Despite all good intentions and preparation by the trainer some factors are beyond the trainer's control. These radically impact on whether a training experience will be positive for participants. Another crucial factor beyond the trainer's control is the role that the manager has in supporting learning in the workplace. Managers and team leaders, who commission training from external trainers, must think about the experience from the participants' perspective. They need both a good experience of training and ongoing reinforcement of the lessons learnt.

The alarm rings for the trainer when participants have been sent on a course with no real idea of what the course is about. Often there will have been no discussion about whether the course fits with their work role. Some staff are even phoned the evening before at home and told to come along. It is not a good start for any trainer to be faced with participants who are not sure why they are sitting in the room. Learning in a workplace environment has to value the participants on the training, and be planned to take account of work demands.

From my experience, managers only think about creating a learning culture and the training and development needs of team members after all the other demands on time. The demands of ensuring that a service meets set performance targets and standards of care while responding to the changing needs of people with dementia makes many managers despair. "How much training does this staff team want?" was a cry from one manager who thought that the one-off training event with an external trainer was enough to meet the team's requirements. Ignoring the training needs of a staff team can lead to stressed, devalued and demotivated workers. Ensuring that a staff team are competent to carry out their role means that the one-off training day is unlikely to change anything other than raise awareness and increase the team members' appetite for more. The challenge is how any training course fits with the ongoing learning culture and leadership practice within the organisation.

Learning acts as a catalyst for change.

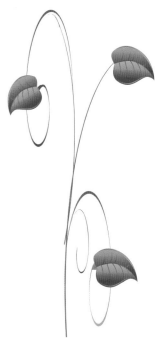

Change happens when teams are led to 'see' and 'feel' the change (Kotter 1995). The vision begins with the manager demonstrating, by their actions, their commitment to the philosophy of care. If that philosophy is person-centred care then a crucial aspect is that the care values also apply to team members. Recently at the dementia centre we have been providing a training course for managers titled 'The manager as leader of dementia practice'. The course helps managers to recognise that their personal leadership style directly influences the culture of learning within their team. One of the five practices of exemplary leadership (Kouzes & Posner 2003) is 'Model the way'. This is about words and actions being consistent. It emphasises that influencing the team begins with the manager or team leader taking time to earn the respect of the team by showing them respect. Many course participants had not made the connection, often because their own line manager had not demonstrated it.

This is the right time for training and it cannot be seen as a luxury. Given the increasing number of people with dementia, there is a need for competent and confident workers. However this has to be a justified confidence (Stephenson 2003). This means that the manager knows that their team member has the right knowledge, value base and skills to do the job. The least cost is the actual training day, as it is what happens afterwards back in the workplace that is critical. The individual worker needs to have confidence in their own knowledge and skills, to have learned from experience, to perform under stress, to

communicate effectively and to collaborate with others. This cannot be achieved unless managers value the training and follow it up.

A conscious and planned effort to shift a team from 'good enough' to 'best' practice also needs the manager to recognise that team members have to be risk takers. This risk is not that of placing someone in danger but rather taking the risk of doing things differently from what has been done before. The manager must be prepared to recognise the importance of supporting team members to be positive risk-takers.

Workplace training cannot be an extra. It has to be part of regular work activity. Too many managers think that the one-off training course with the special external trainer will solve all the problems like magic. All problems of low morale, poor practice and lack of teamwork will be solved by the trainer's toolkit of techniques. In truth, no lasting effect will occur unless there is a follow through after that event which involves team members. Follow through means the manager has to consider how they provide opportunities, as part of the daily work routine, which permit new learning to be tried out in practice. The manager has to own the process of learning.

Kotter JP (1995) *Leading Change*. Harvard Business School Press. Boston, USA.
Kouzes J, Posner B (2003) *Leadership Challenge*. Jossey-Bass, San Francisco.
Stephenson J (2003) Ensuring a holistic approach to work-based learning, in Boud D & Solomon N (eds) *Work-based learning*, Open University Press, Buckingham.

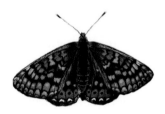

03:11

Time: star or sprint?

Nick Gulliver

Nick Gulliver has worked as a support worker for Dementia Care Partnership, Newcastle for the past seven years, having been a probation officer for the previous 28. He has a BA in social science, a CQSW and MA (History of Ideas). His interests are local history (19th century Newcastle Police Force), campaigning for recognition of a forgotten Tyneside life-saving family, the Craigs, writing and the promotion of reminiscence work with people with dementia

A Jamaican runs the 100 metres in New York. He breaks the world record in less time than it takes to read this sentence. Breathtaking.

A Hubble photograph: at 40 million years old, a 'relatively young' star cluster is some 160,000 light years away in the Large Magellanic Cloud, our near stellar neighbour. Cosmic.

Two images play on my mind. Parking up, I press on towards a weekly appointment. It has been a crowded morning. Visits, a meeting, gossip.

As it is, two images, two metaphors.

The mad dash of the support worker: dementia care's foot soldier. The dreaded half-hour contract in which you are to enter, engage, help raise, wash, dry, cream, shave, dress, prompt meds, feed, clear up, clear away, clear off. And be courteous. And be empathic.

Then, the drive from one end of town to the other in, according to the work roster, nought point nought minutes. If not miraculous, at least exciting.

The man, subject to our ministrations, dealing with the dark matter of his dementia. Lost in inner space, his neurological nebulae inexplicable, exotic, frightening, a minute mirror of the outer universe.

Two times: the busyness of the support worker. The dementia dimension, a fragment of existence withdrawn from Time.

Can there be a meeting of such minds?

Are we not as far apart as athlete from star cluster? Is dialogue – as opposed to two monologues – across our temporal divide possible?

Well, yes. Given a workable passage of time such conversations can and are fruitfully struck up. Even the 30-minute slot is actually no great barrier to such connections, such exchanges of narratives.

The railway historian overlooking the same leafy Gosforth street in which he once lived his idyllic boyhood , whose time at the Royal Grammar School was his memorial time, gradually pieces together the school song last sung in the late '20s, fragment by fragment until, as visit follows Sunday morning visit, enough returns to be sung joyously through.

The Welsh conscientious objector who inexorably forgot his return home, his wife, how to eat, dress, in the end, where to excrete. Whose dementia dimension placed him in his childhood Rhondda; or in a bog behind enemy lines on D-Day where he had been parachuted in as a medic, all but drowned, then captured; or in the post-war Middlesex Probation Service.

Times conjured up as vividly as though yesterday. And, incidentally, an overlap of times, his with mine. My social work observation placement located in the self-same Tottenham Office where he had served a generation before with colleagues mutually remembered. Of such serendipity bonds are formed.

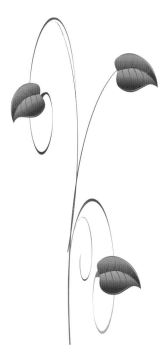

Two memorable memories, two among numerous moments of conviviality with men mostly now deceased. The joy of support work. Optimally, but not necessarily, during those two-, three- or even four-hour domiciliary sessions called 'sit-in services'.

The intimacy of helping strip-naked, bathe, ablute lends itself to recall of sometimes long-forgotten miseries. The Everton apprentice who, homesick, sacrificed professional football for his Geordie familiarities. The scourge of the Scotswood police who, fleet of foot, stole basics – wet fish, potatoes and such like – to tide his mother and brothers over the harsh, fatherless Depression years.

But then, for the sheer multi-layered weavings of time, or rather times (past/present/future; myth/history; memory/primary sources/search station; the unborn/mortality) an exemplary anecdote.

Visiting a 91-year-old retired miner (an ex-pump-man in the Albert, Bleucher and Black Callerton pits). A man hanging on to independence against inevitability. I arrived more animated than usual. I explained that my daughter – recently pregnant – had discovered the launching of the Chilean battle-cruiser 'O'Higgins' at the Armstrong Whitworth Yard for me on Google. I added that this related to my researches into 'The Reid Robbery', a *cause célèbre* in the 1890s when a jewellers was broken into by a group of Chilean sailors.

The nonagenarian Novocastrian interrupted me. "Chinese", said he. "What?" I answered, nonplussed. "Chinamen," he repeated, adding that he had already heard of the case; that his father (also a pitman) had sat him at his knee when he was a small boy to tell him the tale. How a crew of Chinamen had been engaged by Reid's to decorate their shop and how they had secreted gems, trinkets etc piece by piece back to their vessel and had only been apprehended by misfortune. He had heard this when he was about five or six years old around 1918-19 or so, over 80 years before.

No appeal to press and court papers citing only Chileans (Luis Antonuchi, Julien Flores, Josi Tapio and the others) could dissuade him otherwise. Father's word, not written history, was Law, even after so life-long a time. He was not for budging and there was no point trying. Pyjamas on, microwave meal in, we moved on.

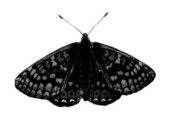

03:12

Different perspectives

Nori Graham

Nori Graham is an Emeritus Consultant in Old Age Psychiatry, Royal Free Hospital, London and former Chairman of the Alzheimer's Society and Alzheimer's Disease International.

Time, with the aid of memory, is the cable that secures us to our past. If we cannot remember when events occurred we cannot make sense of them. Did I start to feel low when my daughter who was visiting me left my room, or did she leave my room because she was so upset by my constant crying? If I cannot remember when, I cannot remember why.

In a similar way it is our sense of time on which our imagination depends when we map our own future. We cannot know when lunch is due if we cannot remember whether we have had our breakfast. If I cannot remember when or even whether an event occurred then I cannot imagine what is going to happen next.

An imagined reverie in a person with dementia:

A lady comes into my room and tells me to get up and get dressed. She is wearing a uniform with a badge on which the word 'Tina' is printed. She then disappears. Some time passes but I cannot work out how much time. Another lady comes in. She has a badge with 'Julie' printed on it. She is obviously angry but I cannot work out why. She also tells me to get dressed and then disappears. I get out of bed and then notice I am wearing my nightie. If I am wearing my nightie it must be time for me to go to bed. I go to bed. Another lady comes in. She is wearing a badge with 'Tina' printed on it. She seems quite angry and starts to get my day clothes out of my wardrobe. Then she starts to dress me, but I can perfectly well dress myself. I can be angry too!

But time can also be an instrument of torture; the need to clock-watch all the time can make us feel persecuted.

Tina's story:

I got up at 6 this morning and I'm not a morning person. I prepared the kids' clothes for school and made breakfast for them and my husband. He arrived back from night shift at 7 and wanted to talk but I didn't have time for that. I woke the boys and dressed them though at 6 and 8 years they really ought to be dressing themselves. I don't have time for that either. I gave them their breakfast as quickly as I could and then took or rather dragged them round to the lady who looks after them before school. Then I went to work arriving around 8.

I have nine residents I have to get ready before they get breakfast at 9. This morning one of them was extremely difficult and resisted being dressed. Breakfast has to be over in 45 minutes because that's when the kitchen staff come in to take the trollies with the dirty crockery away. If they don't take them by 10 they don't have time to get the lunches ready.

By the time the residents have had breakfast and been toileted it's 11 and I can have a sit down with the other staff while the residents watch TV for three quarters of an hour before we get them to the table for lunch. That's the best time of day for me. Yesterday a lady came in and said we ought not to let them watch TV; they weren't being stimulated enough. We ought to use the time better. I expect she's right!

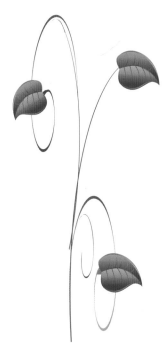

03:13

The stories of my life

Rosas Mitchell

Rosas Mitchell has a background in social work where she has specialised in service development in dementia care. Currently, she works with people helping them record their life stories using both art and therapy. She has been connected to the Dementia Services Development Centre at Stirling for many years.

This is the first day of my life
Languishing on pink chairs
Of cold vinyl
Pushed hard against the wall
Covered in floral tribute
Announcing pattern.

Arm rests nudging
Against nameless neighbours.
A cacophony of sound
Pervades the room
Already impregnated with
Sickly sweet odour.

Mists swirl in
As way points
Fade into obscurity.
Past, present and future
Converging on this moment,
Abstruse and dark.

Is this the first day of my life?
Or is there something else?
Something more?
A key to open the door of my life?

Photos,
Torn and faded,
Small and precious,
Sepia,
Announcing
Familiar faces,
Familiar places.

Pebbles,
Smooth, solid, markings,
Salty flavoured,
Rumbling in response to receding waves,

Patchwork of greens,
Framed in white lace.
Overhead the screech of the oyster catcher
Above the deserted beach.

Memories beckon,
Not well rehearsed actors on a distant stage
But fully present, alive and well,
New dialogues, new perspectives,
A kaleidoscope of stories,
Vibrant and changing.

These are the stories of my life.
I revel in the sense of who I am
Honed for each occasion
A sense of value and worth returned
And dogged determination to move on.

Prickly pear,
Its knobby skin
Lovingly pared,
Revealing succulence,
Orange texture,
Cool and delicious
Tainted with anguish.

Who will listen to the stories of my life?
Who will embrace their repetition?
Who will hear the subtle changes?
Who will magically open the door
To whom I am and what I've been?

Always waking to the first day of my life
And ending with the last
Will be my condemnation

Without you.

Valuing time spent engaging with people

Jackie Pool

Jackie Pool is an occupational therapist and the founder of JPA (Jackie Pool Associates), a UK specialist in care services with particular expertise in dementia.

Some time ago I visited a hospital ward that provided continuing care for people with dementia, where I was working as an occupational therapist. As I came through the door, an obviously harassed nurse-in-charge dashed past me, shouting back over his shoulder: "We haven't had time to do any activities today." There had been some illness amongst the staff team and a new patient had just been admitted, so it was the case that there was a time pressure on those on duty and therefore the basic personal care needs were taking priority.

As an occupational therapist, I am often asked to meet with groups of care home and ward staff to discuss how activity can be a part of care practice. This response of not having time to 'do' activities is very common, understandably, because there is rarely a full complement of staff in our care settings.

We could enter into a debate about why there aren't enough staff, and we may draw the conclusion that if there are insufficient staff then the range of opportunities for engaging in activity must be reduced. However, I think that the conversations I have with some of these groups of staff reveal that it may not be the number of staff available that is always the issue.

If I ask what the members of staff have done with patients or residents up to that point of the day, they are able to describe a range of personal care tasks. Sometimes these are listed as: 'getting them up; toileting them; walking them and feeding them'. This use of language reveals a task-oriented approach to personal care needs, and it seems as though the person as an individual at the centre for receiving this has disappeared!

However, if we use a person-centred approach these tasks become activities to be carried out together with the person with dementia. These activities can now be viewed as "helped John to get up; assisted Enid to use the toilet; supported Jean to walk; enabled Bob and Mary to dine". This is really all about a shift in attitude and doesn't necessarily require any more time to carry out. Instead, the member of staff is now viewing the personal care as an activity with as much value as the traditional leisure activities.

Feedback from many care workers demonstrates that this change of attitude not only benefits their service users but also gives them a higher level of job satisfaction. Now they are no longer "just doing personal care with no time for activities" but they are engaging with services users through 'personal care activities'.

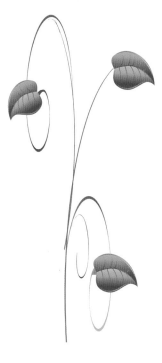

There is time to sing to me

Eva Götell

Eva Götell is a Registered Nurse Tutor and Ph.D. Her thesis 'Singing background music and music events in the communication between persons with dementia and their caregivers in dementia care' was published in 2003. She works as a senior lecturer and a dementia care researcher at Mälardalen University, Sweden.

There was a time when I learned how to take care of myself. Before that I needed people to help me. Nowadays I consider myself to be a decent person. I enjoy looking good, being with people, being nice to them and telling them I enjoy their company.

In the future, there may be a time when I get dementia. At that time, I may well behave in a way that I wish I could prevent. I know I will lose my ability to wash myself, and to understand my environment. I may well behave in a manner that people will experience and call disturbing or problematic. I may not respond to people. I may show agitation, or scream. I may act aggressively or even hit people when they are in close contact with me.

My behaviour might be so difficult that the caregivers, whose help I need for my everyday life, may be stressed themselves. They may find it problematic to meet my needs. I know that they will do their very best and I am sorry that I will probably drive them to the limits of their self-control. Some of them may even lose their temper and behave in an unethical way. I am sorry that these situations may happen. I hope I can act differently when I get dementia, but I may not.

Nowadays researchers are working on finding a medication to cure Alzheimer's disease. There is some success in drugs which slow down the decline and might help people to live an independent life for longer. Unfortunately drugs given for behaviour worsen the condition of people with dementia making them less cognitively able, more likely to fall and worsening their aphasia. Research on nurses' attitudes to disturbing or problematic behaviour is not encouraging; many seem to believe that there is little that can be done.

There is a lot of research on other interventions such as reminiscence therapy, validation therapy, music therapy and dancing showing that they expose the latent skills of people with dementia, helping them to regain their abilities to talk, remember, sing, dance and show improved social skills. It is also claimed that behaviour can improve.

If I get dementia, I tell you right now that I want you to help me to expose the latent skills that I have. Please communicate with me and provide me with enough stimulation that I might act as I used to; being nice to people and telling them I enjoy their company for example. These effects only last for short time and may not last long enough to affect me when you are helping me with more personal tasks such as morning hygiene and getting dressed. I will need other help in finding my latent skills.

I know that caregivers will do their best to help me. They will work to create an understandable world with their talking, their bodies, their movements and their sensory awareness, as well as encouraging me when I have positive or negative emotions and moods. I may, nevertheless, remain confused, have limited speech because of my aphasia and perhaps even lash out or scream. If I do, I will be expressing panic, fear and sadness. My body posture is likely to be slumped and I will be unbalanced when I stand up. I will have little facial expression and eye contact. My skills in washing myself may be very limited perhaps using only one hand, keeping my hand cupped or washing only one side of my body. I may be unable to recognise a toothbrush, a comb or a towel.

And yet, in an inexplicable way, my latent skills can be revealed when the caregivers sing to me while helping me with personal care (Gotell, Brown & Ekman, 2001, 2002, 2003, 2008). If they do this, I will be more cognitively aware, I will understand their verbal language better. I will be less likely to react with resistance, aggression or screaming. I will be more likely to be positive, wanting to participate, show more vitality and positive emotions such as delight, happiness and wonder. My emotional responses will be more positive if caregivers sing with sincerity, warmth, intimacy and vulnerability. Their singing will result in my improved posture and balance. I will have better eye contact and I will be more likely to smile. I may well listen with concentration and perhaps even join in. I may even tell the caregivers that I enjoy the singing or I might comment humorously if they are singing off key. Isn't that amazing?

Their singing may also help me to wash myself, and remember that there are two sides to my body. I may recognise the toothbrush and comb and know how to use them. I may then be able to find my bedroom. Perhaps best of all, while singing the caregivers might experience personal care as easy tasks that enhance their well-being as well as mine.

If I get dementia and I have a damaged brain, in an inexplicable way, my brain will work better for a short time, if caregivers are singing. Right now, all I ask of you if I get dementia, is that you sing for me when you are helping me with personal care. This will not take any extra time, and it will immeasurably improve the experience for both of us.

Brown S, Götell E, Ekman S-L (2001) Music-therapeutic caregiving: The necessity of active-music-making in clinical care. *The Arts in Psychotherapy* 28 (2) 125-135.

Brown S, Götell E, Ekman S-L (2001) Singing as a therapeutic intervention in dementia care. *The Journal of Dementia Care* 9 (4) 33-37.

Götell E, Brown S, Ekman S-L (2002) Caregiver Singing and Background Music in Dementia Care. *Western Journal of Nursing Research* 24(2) 195-216.

Götell E, Brown S, Ekman S-L (2003) The influence of caregiver singing and background music on posture, movement and sensory awareness in dementia care. International *Psychogeriatrics* vol 15 (4) 411-430.

Götell E, Brown S, Ekman S-L (2008) The influence of caregiver singing and background music on vocally expressed emotions and moods in dementia care. *International Journal of Nursing Studies*. Corrected proof online.

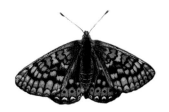

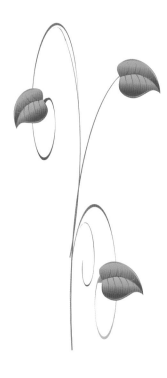

Leaders are closely watched by their constituents and how leaders spend their time is a clear indication of what's really important. If you say that customers and innovation is important to you, ask yourself how much time you're spending time with customers and on driving innovation. People look at how leaders spend their time, as a means to judge if leaders measure up to their talk. Followers ask themselves, 'Does my leader spend time on what they're telling me is important?', 'Do you spend their time on what they say is important?'

You = Your calendar*

*Calendars never lie

All we have is our time. The way we spend our time is our priorities, is our 'strategy'. Your calendar knows what you really care about. Do you?

Tom Peters, management guru
From a presentation on leadership

03:16

Time to read

Jill Manthorpe

Jill Manthorpe is Professor of Social Work and Director of the Social Care Workforce Research Unit at King's College London. She has been involved in dementia research and ageing issues more generally for many years and in addition to studies that are formally commissioned, she has been interested in the portrayal of dementia and ageing in fiction and its relevance to policy, public debate and professional practice. Her current research includes studies of the workforce, safeguarding and mental capacity.

Shortage of time is a fairly constant complaint among those supporting people with a dementia. People with dementia may experience time differently but, for many of us who have tried to support people with dementia, it is not always easy to find the time to see the world from their point of view, or to see how the rest of the world perceives a person with dementia.

This desire, yet also frustration, to move from objective to subjective perspective features strongly in professional training. Time for this is equally pressured but one way of making time more elastic is to think of ways in which personal and professional lives can be bridged in an enjoyable rather than stressful way.

New opportunities to make these imaginative leaps seem to be available, due to the steady increase in fictional accounts of people with dementia and their circumstances. Because reading fiction is one of the nation's major hobbies, especially for women, reading about dementia is likely to be taking place, often by accident. Time spent reading, on the beach or the bus, may be one way of thinking afresh about our own reactions to stories of dementia.

Novels with dementia as a central motif are emerging; but these are small in number. *The Story of Forgetting* by Stefan Merrill Block is one such recent work – spanning the United States in a story of the emergence of a form of early onset dementia, working its way across continents and generations.

So in the peace of a holiday, or the self-constructed quiet bubble of a bus journey, it may be more likely that we come across dementia as a brief mention in everyday reading. Recently, for example, I was enjoying a story of a move to Cornwall when the mother in law of a character turned out to be 'sixpence short of a shilling'. Penelope Lively (1999) deftly drew a picture of an older woman with Alzheimer's disease tyrannised by her family; adding for good measure the evidence from a health visitor's report that misread the situation entirely. In other reading such as crime novels or family sagas, dementia is found – not as a central motif but part and parcel of the lives of many families and communities.

Reading these accounts is very different from newspaper stories of dementia focusing on policy decisions; paying for care or dementia drugs; or the quality of services – or lack of it; or possible new cures.

For some readers, novels about dementia are interesting but often a little exasperating in that they may be magical or otherwise unrealistic. Moreover, it takes a certain compulsive tendency to bring work home with you. Time to read for pleasure may be escapist, in terms of reaching into other worlds, other periods, other emotions.

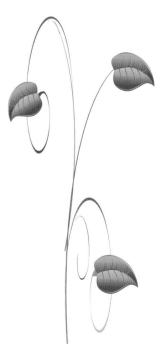

So this is a serendipitous picture. Taking time to read is a way the workforce can look after itself. But along the way we may pick up evidence of a growing familiarity with dementia or Alzheimer's disease that may render our work easier because there is greater recognition. Almost everything that I have read reveals an understanding of the syndrome and the difficulties of managing symptoms. But there is humour too, and most accounts convey sympathy for all concerned.

It may be that such material can be used for training. I think, however, that there is much scope to savour in the space of private reading. If characters with dementia inhabit our imaginative world then this does not turn relaxation into work. It may, however, be a way of picking up ways to reduce the stigma of dementia. Quiet time reading may be a way in which we witness this change.

Lively P (1999) *Spiderweb*. Penguin, London.
Merrill Block S (2008) *The Story of Forgetting*. Random House, London.

What does time mean to you?

In the course of her research in a care home in Yorkshire, England, Claire Craig asked a group of residents what time meant to them. Below are some of the responses:

• *Time is only important to those who need to be somewhere.*

• *They're always asking you about time here, the day, the date, the hour – it's because they think you're a bit mental (taps his finger on his head). I always say the same to the buggers – if you want to know the time buy a watch or better still ask some other bugger.*

• *What do yer want to know the time for. When it's light it's day, when it's dark it's night.*

• *When you get older time doesn't really mean anything – morning, afternoon, day, night – they all look the same.*

• *My mother told me that every year meant another wrinkle and when your face was full you died.*

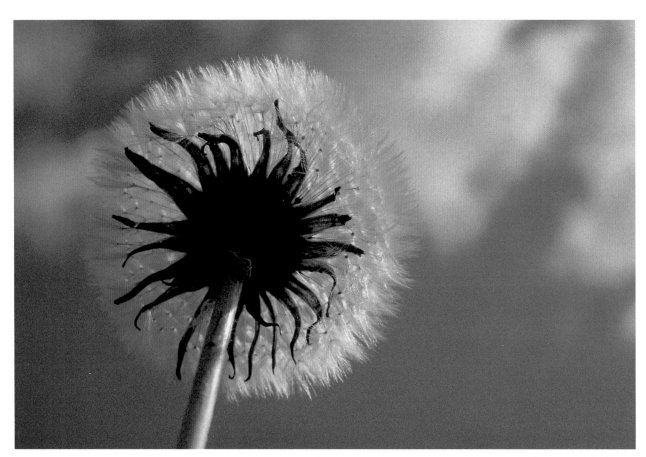

04:00
Clocks

04:01

The unrelenting clock

Patricia Cruse

Patricia Cruse and her husband worked together for most of their married life – 46 years. They had a hotel on Dartmoor and restaurants in Essex and Suffolk. They have two sons and a daughter and six grandchildren. Patricia worked for the Alzheimer's Society for many years and was also a Trustee on the board of Crossroads where she now works full time. Her interest and passion for the care of people with dementia and their carers came about because of her husband's diagnosis of dementia. She has addressed MPs in the House of Commons and given many talks on the role of carers.

Have you ever wondered how we acquired the grand title of 'carer'? I became one, without my knowledge or consent. I thought I was a wife, mother, grandmother, but that did not fit into the scheme of things. I now had to call myself a carer. This title did make me feel uncomfortable as I had not done anything to earn it – or so I thought. However what I found much harder to accept was the gift that went with the title carer: the *unrelenting timepiece*, a clock.

I felt I could manage this new position on my own and by good and careful planning and time management I would not need the help of others. Suddenly time went so much quicker than it did before. If only the clock would slow down a little – I did not do the things I planned to do today, however much I rushed around. But there is respite to look forward to, I hate him going out but I am told I need a break – or do I? I am not sure, his dementia seems so much worse when he comes home (just me thinking it does, probably because I feel guilty). But I will be able to catch up with things while he is away, then we will

be able to spend more valuable time together, my husband and I. Sorry, that cannot be, the clock is getting faster – we need to be together my husband and I, like old times. How long have we got? No one can say.

Is it time to say goodbye? It cannot be, it was only yesterday we painted the bedroom and decided we didn't like the colour – how we laughed. No – please stop the clock, we need some more time, I have still got things to tell him – soppy things, important things. I am sure he still knows me, at least he knows my voice. I am sure.

The clock stopped for him – this moment frozen in time for me. How strange, now the clock has slowed down. How do I fill my days, trying to find something to do to while away the hours? Lying in bed at night and watching the hands on the clock – how slow they move. Another long night and another long day. Then I realise I am no longer a carer so I must give back my *unrelenting timepiece* and move back into the real world and go forward with my memories – he would want that.

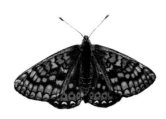

04:02

The CLOX test

Gordon Wilcock

Gordon Wilcock is a Professor of Clinical Geratology at the University of Oxford, UK. He has been involved in the care of people with Alzheimer's disease and other dementias for over 30 years and also in research into these conditions. He was the founder chairman of the UK Alzheimer's Society.

It has long been realised that, although most people consider short-term memory problems to be the main early symptom of Alzheimer's disease, there is also another important area of cognitive impairment. This is known as 'executive function' to which the frontal lobes of the brain make an important contribution. Executive function refers to the thought processes that allow the brain to co-ordinate simple activities and actions to achieve a more complex outcome. For instance, when deciding to bake a cake one has to remember not only what ingredients one needs and also the kitchen implements that are necessary, but also have the ability to put the ingredients together and to use the equipment. This has to be carefully monitored from beginning to end in order to produce something that is edible. Executive function is important for this organisational process. It is often impaired early in Alzheimer's disease, and is also a feature of other dementias.

One of the best ways of measuring this at a simple level is to ask the patient to undertake a CLOX drawing test (Royall *et al* 1998), which is divided into two parts. Each part helps discriminate a failure of executive control from the ability to draw a clock itself i.e. discriminating between executive functions and visuo-spatial and drawing abilities.

The patient is initially asked to draw a clock face setting the hands at, say, 1:45 in such a way that even a child could read the time from the final drawing. The patient is presented with a blank piece of paper and a pencil or pen, and has to decide the size of their drawing, remember to distinguish between a digital or analogue representation, work out where to position the clock on the piece of paper, remember to put in the numbers in a logical order and to space them equally, draw the hands and distinguish between the hour and the minute hand, decide what sort of numerals to employ etc. This involves quite a lot of thought processing and monitoring of performance as well as memory, even though it seems an essentially simple task. Their performance is then scored.

The next step is to ask the patient to copy a clock that the examiner draws while the person is watching. The patient's attempt to copy the clock is then scored in a similar way to their initial attempt, and the scores compared. It is therefore possible to detect whether an initial inability to undertake the task satisfactorily is due to problems with executive function, and if so how bad it is, or whether it represents different problems in undertaking drawing tasks for whatever reason.

This test only takes a few minutes and is a valuable adjunct to other tests that are used to examine memory function. It is important to remember, however, that this ability (executive function) is affected by a number of different illnesses as well as Alzheimer's disease, such as a significant level of depression, Parkinson's disease and other conditions affecting the brain.

Royall DR, Cordes JA, Polk M (1998) CLOX: an executive clock drawing task. *Journal of Neurology, Neurosurgery & Psychiatry* 64:588-594.

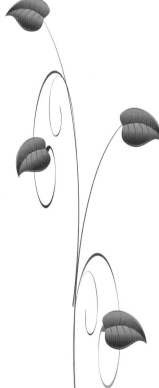

04:03

Body clocks

Annie & Ricky Pollock

Annie Pollock established Arterre Landscape Consultancy in 1987 and specialises in design for frail elderly people and people with dementia. She lectures on external design at Heriot Watt University, and on external environments for people with dementia at international conferences as well as for the Dementia Services Development Centre (DSDC) at Stirling University. She has written a booklet for the DSDC on Garden Design for People with Dementia, based on her award winning show garden for Alzheimer Scotland at the Royal Horticultural Show in Scotland (1999), and is Director of Landscape Design at the DSDC.

Richard Pollock founded the architectural and planning consultancy Burnett Pollock Associates (BPA) in Edinburgh 1974. Since then, BPA has established both design and research expertise in sustainable development, specialised care accommodation, assistive technology for disabilities and dementia friendly design. Richard is also the Director of Architecture at the Dementia Services Development Centre at the University of Stirling, has lectured widely and authored several research papers including writing and editing the DSDC publications 'Designing Interiors for People with Dementia' and 'Designing Lighting for People with Dementia'.

Working at the Dementia Services Development Centre at the University of Stirling, we are using and developing the design audit tool (DSDC 2009), and undertaking design consultancies. As a result, we spend a lot of time in care homes throughout the UK, watching what goes on while we look at the building design and talk to the management.

We have the impression that the daily routine in most care homes is very similar:

- From about 9pm to about 9am, the focus is the bedroom – people are expected to be asleep or in their beds.
- About 10am, after breakfast, there is usually some planned activity, which winds down to a lunch about midday.
- Lunch takes about 40 minutes and then there is a quiet period.
- There is usually some planned activity in the middle of the afternoon, and then another lull before the evening meal at about 6pm.
- Nothing organised happens after that except a nightcap for those still up at about 8.30pm.

Also we realise that problems of sleep disturbance at night are common and the reasons for this may include medications, physical problems, social setting, and psychological conditions. An alternative to medication had recently has been tried with some success, although such research studies are still very preliminary. Healthy elderly patients were given a timed exposure to bright light in the evening, resulting in improved sleep patterns with less wakefulness in the night (NSF Centre for Biological Timing). We are both strong advocates of easy access to the outdoors, where daylight levels are exponentially stronger than average interior lighting. Being able to go outside may also contribute in many other ways to a person's health and well-being.

We have begun to be very interested in the 'circadian rhythm' or 'biological body clock', and are aware that people may have very different daily rhythms. We ourselves have strong body clocks: Ricky is what Dr Hastings (2009) calls a 'lark', rising early and at his best in the morning, whereas Annie is an 'owl', preferring to have a leisurely start, yet often working late at night. We know that circadian rhythms are influenced by a lot of things – including daylight and age – and that there are dips during the day when mental and physical performance are low.

We are currently developing a visual way of noting the 24-hour 'body clock', which would be useful not only in understanding individual body rhythms, the 'lark' or the 'owl' – but would also be a simple graphic way of noting the results of research such as that described above.

The challenge is in developing a simple clock graphic, that is easy to use, that can not only show a care home routine, but also be used to show the 'body

clock' of each resident. It would then be very easy to spot where there is a lack of fit.

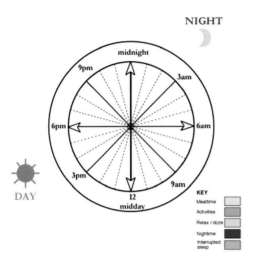

TEMPLATE FOR THE 'BODY CLOCK'

This template (currently under development) is for a 24-hour clock that could be filled in easily by anyone with a pack of colour pencils.

By filling in each segment with the appropriate colour to show the activity being undertaken at that time of the day, an activity pattern can be visually portrayed.

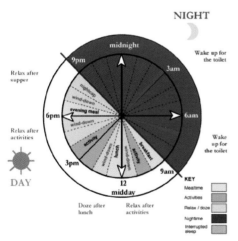

TYPICAL DAILY ROUTINE IN MOST CARE HOMES
shown in 24 hour 'Body Clock' format

In this example, the Body Clock template has been filled in to show the typical routine seen in many care homes, as noted above.

Approximately half the day is seen as 'night', i.e. to be spent in the bedroom, and the 'awake' hours are punctuated by meals, activity and rest.

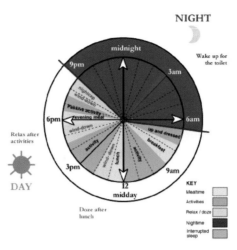

BODY CLOCK FILLED IN FOR THE 'LARK'

Here, the Body Clock is filled in to show a typical day for the 'Lark', and it is immediately visible that this body rhythm requires less sleep and gets going a lot earlier in the morning than the care home example.

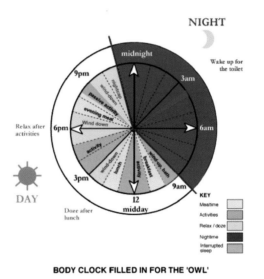

BODY CLOCK FILLED IN FOR THE 'OWL'

Lastly, the 'Owl' – who rises later and goes to bed later also.

This tool could also be used to undertake research, for example on those taking medication, those with sleep problems etc., and to compare whether there are any changes, for example if these people had a greater exposure to more strong light and/or daylight and outdoor activity.

For a person with dementia, this body clock diagram would need to be completed by someone who knows him or her well.

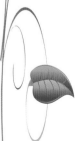

Ideally it would be best if it were done by the person himself or herself, before or shortly after diagnosis. We hope that if we can develop this template into a really simple diagrammatic tool, it could be made easily available to anyone considering moving into 'long stay' care, and updated regularly to take account of changes such as through illness or medication.

We are working on this tool which we hope can be electronic in due course, in the hope that it will enable us all – managers, staff, residents, family and friends – to structure the care home routines to respond better to each individual's body clock.

Dementia Services Development Centre (2009) Design for people with dementia: audit tool.
Hastings M (2009) Interview on *Horizon*, BBC2, 24 February 2009.
NSF Centre for Biological Timing at the University of Virginia. Biotiming tutorial.

How long is an hour

William Purcell

After working as a fireman and an IT manager, William Purcell is now a housekeeping assistant in Adams House residential dementia unit which is run by CrossReach.

How long is an hour for Jenny
Sitting all day in her chair
Not moving a muscle just staring
As the minute hand ticks, ticks away.

04:05

Clocks

Mary Marshall

Miss Turnbull used to get up in the small hours of the night and walk about her care home. It was assumed that she had lost her sense of time with her dementia. She caused disruption to the night staff and seemed thoroughly bewildered. A care assistant found a large faced clock and put it beside her bed. Miss Turnbull started to get up at the normal time.

A third of older people report fair or poor eyesight. Given that most people with dementia are older, they will have the same degree of impaired vision. The problem for people with dementia is that they are often unable to understand that their eyesight is failing and they are also unable to take action to compensate for this.

Clocks are a long established technical aid, which we all rely on to keep us in tune with everyone else in terms of when things are happening. In any situation where we need to be doing something with someone else, we use time as shown by a clock (or watch) as a way of synchronising our activities.

Yet we often fail to understand that many older people cannot see clocks properly. A lot of modern clocks are very hard to read if you have impaired eyesight. They do not have clear numbers, they are often too small and the hands do not always point clearly at the numbers. For older people with a degree of cognitive impairment a digital clock can be incomprehensible. We no longer have chiming clocks in our homes – these can be very helpful if you have difficulty seeing or understanding the clock. The problems are even more serious at night. Luminosity is often insufficient. The clocks on the bedside table are usually small. Is it surprising that people with dementia get up at the wrong time and sometimes even put their clothes on and go outside? This is always blamed on the dementia, which is only partly the case.

So what do we do about it? The ideal night-time clock does not exist. It would have a large, well-lit analogue face beside an indicator showing am or pm and the day of the week. This kind of clock does exist with digital numbers but this is not understandable by many people with dementia.

Mr Forsyth was an ex-engineer who knew he had a problem with clocks at night. He understood digital clocks and was much helped by a clock that projected the time on to the ceiling. Whenever he woke up, he was able to see the clock. Mrs Clark's son put a similar one into his mother's bedroom but it was of no use because she did not understand the numbers.

Until a suitable clock becomes available, there are some interim solutions. One is a large, analogue clock near a low light.

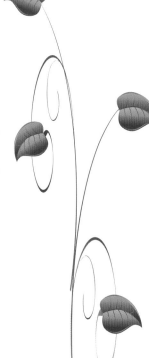

Another is a movement detector near the bed, which switches on a low light to illuminate the clock if the person sits up. Some people, like Mrs Turnbull, simply need a larger bedside clock because they are able to turn the bedside light on.

Large, clear, illuminated analogue clocks should be the first piece of technology tried when a person with dementia seems to be losing their sense of time. Some may need a chiming clock. For many people this will be all they need.

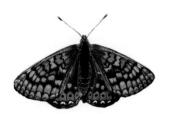

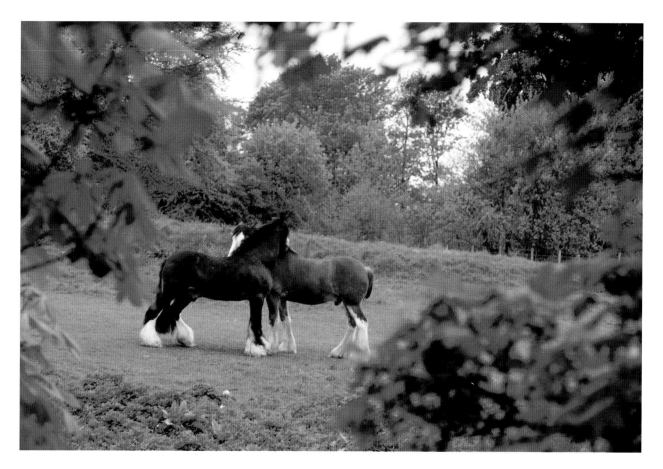

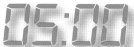

Time to love

05:01

'When do you go back?'

Philip Hurst

Philip Hurst is Policy Manager at Age Concern England – a role which combines both influencing national health policy and interpreting policy as it relates to older people. He previously worked in a range of management posts in the NHS. His contribution is written in a personal capacity.

"When do you go back?" My dad recalls with clarity the first question he was always asked when coming home on leave as a young soldier in the second world war. Not quite the question he was hoping to be asked, or the time he wanted to focus on.

The same question is now put to me, this time from my mum, on my visits 'home'. The questions are infrequent at first but, as the date of my leaving draws closer, they are repeated more often, as if my mum knows the time is close but can't quite retain when it actually is.

Two calendars seem to be a source of great reassurance. One, a gift from holiday from an aunt many years ago, is turned daily to reveal the new date. That is the anchor and helps with reference to the other calendar, a month-by-month wall calendar on which key dates and appointments are written. Not too different from the way most of us use calendars and diaries really, but mum checks this second calendar repeatedly, especially when she isn't occupied with something else.

But just as the calendars are helpful in making sure that things are not forgotten, the actual time of appointments, events and, in my case, train departures, is a source of anxiety. In many ways this is not new. Mum has always wanted to 'make sure we are in good time'; it is just that now things are taken to a greater extreme – of being ready hours in advance, wanting to leave far too early, and worrying about being late. Delaying tactics have only limited success, so we set off 'in good time' to arrive early and wait. At which point mum will happily tell us that we needn't have set off so early! In the end we can still laugh at this, if not learn from it. I know that things will change but, for the time being, there's a pleasing certainty that the first question to face me next time I visit will be: "When do you go back?"

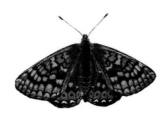

05:02

A carer's personal journey over time

Patricia Burns

Patricia Burns, 72, was until 10 years ago a happy contented wife, mother and homemaker. Life changed when her husband, Tom, was diagnosed with Parkinson's disease and as his health deteriorated he became more and more dependent on her. This is how Patricia became a carer 'by chance'. In 2000 a diagnosis of dementia added to Tom's dependence and Patricia tirelessly and passionately cared for him, honouring his wish to die at home with his family around him. Patricia and Tom had many hurdles to cross and it is why Patricia has a passion to share her journey in order that it might help others along the 'caring pathway'.

A carer is a person who happens into the position by chance. As a consequence a carer needs time to adjust and to open up and not be afraid to ask the questions that need to be asked, so they can get the answers they need to make the caring role much easier.

If I had to define the term, I would say a carer is someone who:

- takes responsibility for the welfare of another person
- develops a strong personality and knows how to speak up for themselves and others
- gathers information and then knows how to put that information to good use
- learns the terms that best describe their loved one's condition, so they can discuss these issues with health professionals
- understands and has compassion for the person they are caring for
- is dedicated to the one they are caring for
- is emotionally attached to their responsibilities as a carer
- makes sacrifices willingly
- looks after another person as well as themselves
- displays a sense of humour
- is a positive thinker
- always looks ahead
- wants to make a difference
- should be valued
- is vital to the future of the health care system.

What a difference there would be for those people needing to be cared for if these qualities could be recognised.

My role as a carer was to take care of my husband and to keep him as well as I could for as long as I could.

Looking back on my caring role I wish there had been a manual for me to follow, although I am not sure how it would work, as everyone is different!

Over time I have learned a lot. I'm sure I have forgotten as much as I can still remember.

If I spend time to reflect on the past ten years of my husband's illness it leaves me very sad and devastated to have watched my loved one, slowly in so many ways, become a childlike dependant.

So I resist instead and turn my thoughts to a time when my husband was still able to travel this beautiful country we live in. It is my time to reflect on the wonderful places we have visited, the concerts we attended and all the beautiful people who came into our lives because of my husband's illness, not in spite of it.

I never thought, for one minute in time,

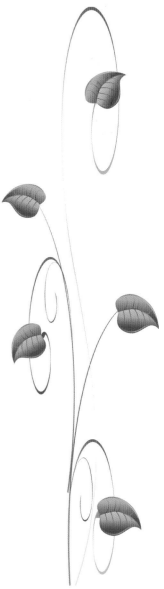

that my caring role would end; but end it did. At that point in time I realised that I had put all my energy into caring for my husband and I did not plan for my life when the job was done.

What would I do now? I kept hearing the words "take care of the carer". Along the way I thought I knew what this meant; now I am not so sure. Maybe now I will have the time to explore this time in my life and work out what it means!

I have discovered that writing down my story has helped me greatly to work through the issues I should have dealt with along the way.

Carers should try to make a plan for their own well-being. I know this is not always easy. Consider making time for yourself by accessing some respite, even if it is only a few hours a week. Maybe this decision should be encouraged early in the caring role.

This is the one thing I did not do and I wish I had. Remember "take care of the carer". I have asked myself, time and time again, did I...

- take care of myself?
- make sure that I got enough sleep to stay well and carry on?
- take time out to recharge the batteries?

- give myself permission to be angry? Maybe I said or did something I felt bad about. I now need to be kind to myself and remember carers are not perfect!
- allow myself a day off?
- heed the warnings of stress?
- accept the offer of respite?
- ask for help in the last 10 years of my husband's illness?

I was sure I could do it all. My husband wanted to stay at home and I could not let him go. I thought I could do it all.

Time is the one thing that carers do not have to spare. I think in hindsight if I had been able to find a few minutes to write down this story as it happened it would have been a great help to me. I wish I had done this. I wish I could still remember the good, the bad and the interesting things that happened to my husband over the timeframe of his illness. I wish there was a hall of fame for all the beautiful people who helped my husband and me to make our journey so much easier than it could have been.

I will take this opportunity to say thank you to all the wonderful people who gave me the tools to work with and to those who contributed to the care and welfare of my husband and my family.

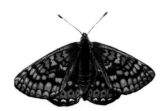

05:03

A question of balance

Brian Lawlor

Brian Lawlor is the Conolly Norman Professor of Old Age Psychiatry at St James's Hospital and Trinity College, Dublin.

When I reflect on the meaning of time in dementia, I think first and foremost of the time spent caring and the lack of time for oneself when you are a caregiver. I am instantly reminded of the title of Nancy Mace and Peter Rabins' book, *The 36 hour day* (2006) which embodies for me the magnitude of the caregiving task and the sense of endlessness and disruption of the normal circadian cycle of life and living that caring in dementia can involve. The time spent needs time for self in return, a balancing of the books, if the caregiver is to achieve the goal of successful caregiving. That is where we as clinicians need to focus more of our time and effort to enable a state of time equilibrium to exist for the caregiver where there are no large time debts to pay back.

Mace N, Rabins P (2006) *The 36 hour day.* Johns Hopkins University Press, Baltimore.

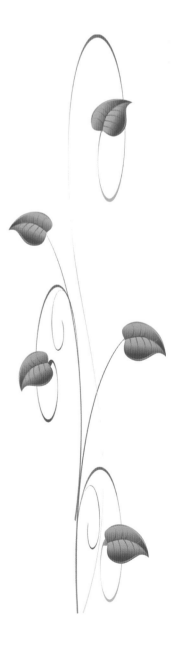

Time together

Ingrid Hellström & Mike Nolan

Ingrid Hellström, PhD, RN, has a background in gerontological nursing. She is a Senior Lecturer at Ersta Sköndal University College, Stockholm, Sweden. Her main research interest is older people with dementia and their spouses.

Mike Nolan is Professor of Gerontological Nursing at the University of Sheffield. He has long-standing interests in the needs of family carers and of vulnerable older people in a range of care environments, and has published extensively in these areas.

Time together captures the importance of being a 'couple' to Lisa and Carl Eriksson, who participated in a longitudinal interview study in Sweden between 2001-2006. The aim of the study was to explore the ways in which older people with dementia and their spouses experience dementia over time, especially the impact it has on their interpersonal relationships and patterns of everyday life (Hellström et al 2007). Lisa and Carl were one couple of the 20 who took part, with Lisa being interviewed six times and Carl five. Carl had dementia.

Lisa and Carl had spent most of their time together since they first met at a party in 1949. At the time of the first interview they had been married for over 50 years and had two daughters, who were living with their families in another part of Sweden and were therefore unable to provide direct support on a daily basis.

Lisa and Carl relied on each other in all aspects of their daily lives. They had lived, for almost 30 years, in a semi-detached house with a nice garden, which was Lisa's pride and joy. Each spring they both tried to find the first forget-me-not of the year in their garden for their partner. This reflected their enduring love and affection for each other with Carl noting "we like to be together and we understand each other in the best way".

However, 15th August 2001 proved a turning point in their lives, as Carl was diagnosed as having Alzheimer's disease. Lisa never forgot this day and initially she was very sad and "cried inside", unable at first to show her feelings to her husband. However, over time they started to be more open with each other and talked about the impact of the condition on their shared lives. They took one day at the time and tried to adjust to their new situation. They had initially planned to move closer to one of their daughters, but later thought it better to stay in their familiar surroundings, so that Carl could find his way about the house and in the neighbourhood. Their world became smaller when Carl was forced to stop driving, and they had to walk to the shops. At first Carl accompanied his wife, but he started to get very nervous among people and preferred to sit outside the mall, waiting for his wife. When she had finished the shopping, he helped to carry the provisions home.

In common with many couples in the study Carl and Lisa didn't look to the future but rather lived for today. Each night before she went to sleep Lisa used to decide what they were going to do the following day, or as Carl put it: Lisa "has to run the business now". Despite a gradual decline in Carl's cognitive ability the couple remained close with small rituals gaining increasing significance. Lisa would ask if she was not there "who is going to go to put the blanket around him in the evening?", and told how Carl used to hold her hand when going to sleep; he wanted to be close to her. He would follow her with his eyes when she moved around in the home and in the garden. Lisa did not find this distressing for, as Carl said, "I have my wife close by all the time".

Eventually time began to have a different meaning. Carl started to attend a day care centre for people with dementia and, although he enjoyed this, Lisa felt that she had let him down. Carl had increasing difficulty in grasping time. He was always in a hurry, afraid of missing the bus to the centre. Consequently he was dressed and ready to go several hours before the bus was going to pick him up.

At the time of the last interview in 2006, Lisa was widowed. She telephoned and said that her husband had passed away and that she was interested in telling us about their last time together. We visited her shortly after the funeral and she told us that Carl had been acutely ill one evening, and she called an ambulance. He was admitted to hospital and stayed there for nearly two weeks. Lisa hardly left his side during his illness. He never recovered and he passed away very peacefully one night with his wife and two daughters at his side. After his funeral Lisa was looking through his clothes and she said that she was going to keep all his ties, as during his life Carl had taken great care with his appearance. Carl's collection of ties became her "ties to their past".

Hellström I, Nolan M, Lundh U (2007) Sustaining 'couplehood'. Spouses' strategies for living positively with dementia. *Dementia* 6 383-409.

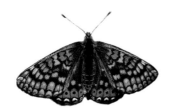

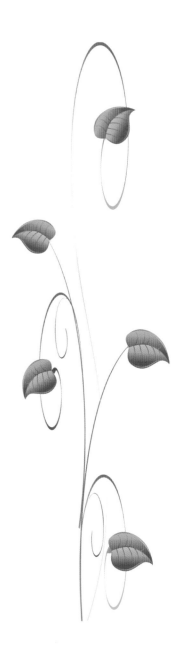

05:05

Time and memory

Kirsty Bennett

Kirsty Bennett is an architect who has designed and researched environments for people with dementia over many years. She has also volunteered as a caregiver, and more recently helped care for her mother. She currently works for the Uniting Church in Victoria and Tasmania as Manager Major Projects and Architecture.

In my experience, there is a lot of sadness associated with dementia: for the person themselves, for their family, and for their friends as the dementia progresses. But there can also be precious gifts, moments when a person is no longer limited by practicalities and loses the limitations that often face the rest of us. We can be given a glimpse of a different way of seeing things, of something special, something that we otherwise may never see.

It seemed to me that when my Mum had Alzheimer's, time no longer had to be linear. There didn't have to be a distinction between what happened when she was 20 and what happened when she was 70. She could move from one era to another with ease. It did not matter that her daughter of 40 could not have been there when she herself was only 20.

I remember one night, as it was getting dark, Mum looked outside and lamented that her father had not come to see her. I knew that he had been dead for over 50 years, and if he was alive would have been about 110! But for her, at that moment, he was 50, she was 20 again, and she longed for him to come and she expected him to come.

This was first of many conversations about my grandfather. And over the coming months, I heard more about this man that I had never met, than I had in the 40 years before. And it was not so much in the stories she told me, or what she remembered, but the way she remembered that made such an impression on me. Her love for him shone through. And I gained a sense of this person that had obviously been so special to her and so important in her life, although she had only been 26 when he had died.

Without dementia, I doubt that this ever would have happened. The past was a long time ago and the memories had faded. But because time was no longer linear, Mum could unknowingly give me a glimpse of my grandfather, a glimpse that was rich and full of love, with emotion that said more than words ever could. Indeed a precious gift.

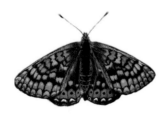

05:06

Past, present and future

Barbara Pointon

Barbara Pointon MBE lectured in music at Cambridge until she took early retirement to care for her husband, Malcolm – a 16-year journey documented in ITV's Malcolm and Barbara... Love's Farewell (2007). She is an Ambassador for the Alzheimer's Society and campaigns internationally for a better deal for people with dementia and their carers.

When my husband Malcolm, after 16 years of living with Alzheimer's, died at the age of 66, kind friends consoled me with, "But the real Malcolm died ages ago!" But did he?

Sure enough, over time, Malcolm had lost all the things the world values: his job, social life, piano-playing, recognition of family members, mobility, speech, physical functions – the list could go on – and I truly mourned each loss. But the real Malcolm, his very essence (identity, spirit, call it what you will) was there right to the end and love lives on.

This poem was written several years ago in an Alzheimer's Society conference workshop on creative writing, where we were asked to write a message to someone important to us, and I remember the words just tumbling out:

To Malcolm

You weren't always like this.

Your hands lie still and limp,
Yet once those fingers flew over the piano keys.

Your eyes stare vacantly ahead,
Yet once you saw pictures in the clouds.

Your legs twitch, dangling useless from the hoist,
Yet once you strode for miles, untiring.

Your voice is silenced.

Yet once you handled words with mastery –
for the BBC, for your students,
for the drama group, ad infinitum.

Your arms have lost their strength,
Yet once you held me in passionate embraces.

But you
Are still you
And I will love you – always.

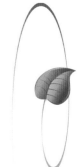
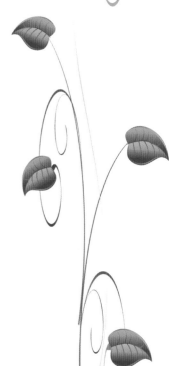

71

05:07

Draughts

Barbara Bowers

Barbara Bowers is a Professor of Nursing at the University of Wisconsin-Madison in the US. For 25 years she has been a researcher in long-term care and has taught students who are interested in careers caring for older adults. As a young child she was fortunate to have several grandparents and great-grandparents in her life.

Some memories endure… reappearing unbeckoned and unexpected. They come with strong emotions, with sounds and scents of their own.

Cherry pipe tobacco… a dark blue pipe cleaner stained brown with use… a finger tapping on the stuffed bowl of a pipe, a clock chiming the hour… and the half hour… the soft, slow, husky, well worn voice of an old man… the scent of 'old man'. The Lennon Sisters singing 'Shake me I rattle, Squeeze me I cry'.

I loved to hear his stories about the boy growing up on a farm in Iowa... They say his memory is going.

I marvel at the stories he has to tell, how well he remembers them, how he can tell the same story over and over without losing a single detail.

A wooden draughtboard sits between us… between me and my great grandfather, George… set on the green card table with the wobbly legs. I feel queasy, even now, recalling the green leather, spinning stool… my favourite place to sit… sneaking a forbidden spin…

Waiting for him to take his turn. He moves black… I move red.

Puffing and tapping on his pipe. I watched his hand move the black pieces, the wrinkled, yellow skin, covered with a maze of dark blue lines. I touched the dark blue lines... just to see what they felt like. He didn't mind.

I felt comforted, loved, secure… undisturbed by the knowledge of what was to come.

Always comforting, always welcome… this Memory.

Another clock chiming the hour… and the half hour. Not the same chime but the same regularity…the same marker of passing time. Now cigarette smoke, without the sweetness of cherry tobacco.

A rattling cough disturbing the silence… An old man… my father… A draughtboard, now plastic… with red and black pieces… set on a white linen table cloth… on a sturdy and expertly crafted walnut dining table.

The table came to me when my father began 'to fail' and moved into our home.

The linen tablecloth was my mother's treasure… then used only on special occasions… now stained from constant, loving use.

A simple game… not as complicated as many games we had played together in the past. Newly without the excitement of political debates.

Mostly now in silence… broken by the exhaling of smoke, a cough… and the chiming of a clock…marking the passing of time.

Waiting… waiting… Will he move? Has he fallen asleep? Has he lost the ability to play this simple game? Hands poised over the board, yellow, blotchy skin with dark blue lines running along the back of his hands. I trace the dark blue lines with my eyes. Finally a move. A good move. He smiles… pleased with himself. I feel relieved, comforted, loved, secure… this time disturbed by the sadness of knowing what is to come. I push that thought away but it's not gone.

He moves black. I move red.

The mingling scents of beach, pine forest and extinguished camp fire. Flies buzzing.

Waves spill onto the beach with no sound at all. A draughtboard sits on a picnic table covered with a plastic red and white table cloth. The board tilts, sitting on the not-quite-even table top warped from years outside in the damp. The draughtboard sits between us… between me and my grandchildren… Daisy and George…

They take red. I take black.

05:08

For auction

Davis Coakley

Professor Davis Coakley is Professor of Medical Gerontology at Trinity College Dublin and a consultant physician at St. James's Hospital. He is a founder of the Dementia Services Information and Development Centre in Ireland and has written a number of books on medical history and a biography of Oscar Wilde.

Tarnished silver,
Trinkets,
Ornaments in brass,
An inlaid writing box.

And on the wall
A photograph –
Of father and his son –
A monochrome in brown.

Underneath,
Three words
In faded ink
'Katherine, remember us'.

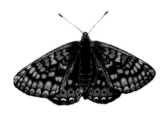

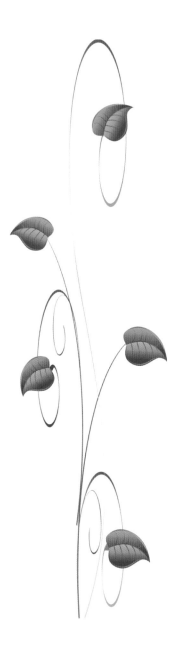

05:09

Time to reflect

Elaine White

Elaine White is a Registered Nurse and currently a permanent part-time Educator for Alzheimer's Australia NSW. Elaine has a passion about best practice in aged and dementia care. She has a wealth of experience in problem solving complex and challenging situations with a focus on enhancing the quality of life for people living with dementia.

Dementia is a thief of time; it may strip the person's time to grow old together with their lifelong partner, it may prevent them taking that overseas trip as planned, it may make them unable to recognise their grandchildren or family members. There are lots of negatives to reflect on but we should not waste our energies on the things we cannot change but rather concentrate on the positives.

However, there needs to be time to become accustomed to the diagnosis of dementia. Time to digest how terminal a diagnosis it is and what the future may encompass. A time for grieving for both the person diagnosed with dementia and their carers; time to talk through all the options and set directions in place for future planning.

As carers, our greatest gift is that of time. We need to give our time to step into the person's 'world of dementia' and share their life's joys and sorrows. For the person living with dementia it is a world that has robbed them of clarity of thinking – their short-term memory has gone but long-term memory is still intact.

It is therefore a time to listen to, focus on and celebrate the person's life achievements, share their stories and the many roles the person has had:
• Son/daughter, grandchild and sibling
• Friend, student, employee and colleague
• Boyfriend/girlfriend, lover, fiancé and spouse/partner
• Parent, neighbour, citizen, confidant, grandparent and senior citizen.

It is a time to appreciate the intertwining of these roles, stepping in and out of them as the time goes by. Be inspired by the person's experience and wisdom gained along the way; the impact they may have had on others. Time to understand the experiences that have contributed to making up the sum total of the 'who' the person is today.

Make the most of the time left, precious time to share feelings, unspoken feelings of long ago. Time to validate the person's worth. Time to laugh over past pleasures and cry together for past losses or mistakes. Time spent to acknowledge regrets and disappointments and/or hostilities can be so worthwhile, allowing the person to express their unspoken love, resolve some old conflicts and/or attend to unfinished business.

When the journey becomes rough and residential care may be the best alternative, it is not the end, it is time though for a carer to let go; let someone else do the caring and the carer do the loving.

Finally enjoy the days together, no matter where the person living with dementia is, love, live old memories and laugh together. Never underestimate the power of laughter, it gets us through many a difficult time.

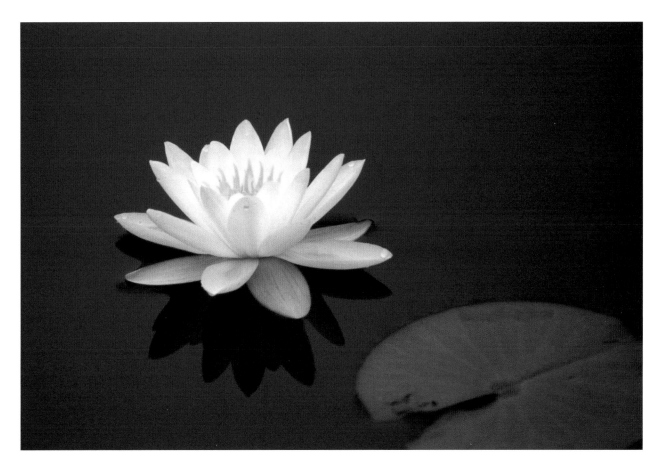

06:00

Being in the moment

06:01

Spending time, enjoying time

Stephen Judd

Dr Stephen Judd is the Chief Executive of Hammond Care, an independent Christian charity that exists to improve the quality of life of older people in need through providing care and services both in the community and in residential facilities. Hammond Care specialises in dementia services and has a particular commitment to the financially disadvantaged.

I ran up the steps two at a time. I was 30 minutes late for a meeting with the lawyers. We were taking over an organisation and we had to flatten things immediately; I had missed a meeting with my own executive staff, and in five minutes was supposed to be simultaneously at Hammondville. I foolishly had not eaten breakfast that morning – no time – and was now starving. In my pocket my phone began to demand my attention.

The day, which in my PDA calendar had been so carefully itemised and seemingly manageable, had been lost to me. I was outta time.

Forty minutes later I was speeding along the motorway towards Hammondville, where, amongst other things, my calendar told me I was to meet with staff about the future of our arts therapy programme in Southwood, one of our dementia-specific nursing homes.

My colleagues were held up. So, winning back time, I wandered down to Southwood. I rang the doorbell of Kalina, a small domestic cottage. It was answered by a smiling Jane, a staff member, "Hi Stephen, good to see you. Come on in. Would you like a cuppa? No, you sit down. I'll get it."

As I sat in the lounge room I was surprised to find that I was slowing down. My neck and shoulder muscles had been tense: now they were relaxing. I watched the routine of the cottage. Fred was walking out to the garden, watering can in hand; Mary was helping in the kitchen; Doris was dusting and rearranging some decorative china; while Bill, once a maitre d' and still, it seemed, in charge, was eyeing the plates and cups and glasses and picking up used plates and glassware, taking them to the kitchen and rearranging the table settings. Peter was snoring faintly in his favourite chair. It was just a regular post-lunch scene, really. Joyce came out of her room, looked at me quizzically and, after my brief introduction, sat opposite me. She observed me cautiously.

Jane brought me a cup of tea. I take it black and none; it was white and sweet. I drank it anyway. Joyce smiled: I was deemed 'okay'.

A minute passed, then five. I sat. Time had slowed and, then, seemed to stop.

It seemed like I was in Kalina Cottage for ages. In fact, it was less than an hour. Some hours later, as I drove on the motorway with the setting sun behind me, I reflected on the evening ahead. A quick bite in front of the telly, and then I will have to work on those three Government reports. They were marked 'Draft' but I know it will be hard to change or amend. Why do they give you so little time? Maybe they don't really want my opinion!

As the traffic crawls into Harbour Tunnel and my patience is being lost, my neck and shoulders are tensed again. Suddenly, without warning, a saying of my father pops out of the deep recesses of my mind: "Beware the barren-ness of a busy life!"

Dammit, he's right. I inch forward into the darker tunnel. I think of the people I have left at Kalina Cottage. I think of their sense and use of time and think, "I reckon maybe they've got it right! I am certainly spending time but am I enjoying it?". A cruel thought blurts into my head; do I have to wait for the onset of dementia to enjoy my time here? I laugh out loud, so much so that the person next to me in the traffic gives me a look.

06:02

Every Wednesday morning

Marie Mills

Marie Mills is a researcher and chartered psychologist, specialising in psychotherapy and group work with people who have had a diagnosis of dementia, and who are aware that they have memory problems.

The memory support group for people with dementia begins on time, at 10.30am to be precise. Members trickle in prior to this. As Grace is handed a cup of coffee and invited to choose a biscuit, she says, "This is wonderful! Such a welcome! I must say it is a very unexpected pleasure at my time of life." She says this every week, but her enjoyment and sense of belonging always seem newly minted. Time coalesces in the midst of such structured time. It is the paradox of dementia where time has both profound and little meaning.

As a group we begin to idly talk about the present, who is not here today, and the reasons why. Current news is briefly discussed but we are drawn more towards past memories, achievements and experiences which excite interest, admiration and often sympathy. We jointly reflect on lives well lived and the shared telling becomes a narrative – a timeless narrative. We are listeners to the narrator, and as such we climb mountains, experience Iraq as a beautiful place with gentle kindly people, converse with the Queen, fly damaged planes in World War Two and know the fear of crashing behind enemy lines. We revisit old schools and introduce our teachers, respected or hated, to a new audience. Past careers, which offer a strong sense of identity, are modestly explained. The life achievements in the group are staggering and instil awe. In the moment this is reflected back to the narrator. We see self-esteem begin to unfurl. It is not dead but has been undernourished.

We touch on the present, the importance of these memories and marvel at their decades of endurance. With humour, we share our forgetfulness and, while insight lasts, we mourn the burden it places on those who care for us. We tell one another that this illness is no one's fault and one day there will be a cure. In the meantime we have each other. Grace says, "It is a huge consolation to know you are not alone with this Alzheimer's." The group agree silently with nodding heads… it is a timeless moment.

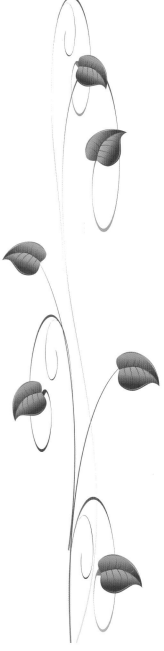

06:03

The passing of time

Graham Stokes

Graham Stokes is Director of Dementia Care for Bupa Care Services. His interests are neuropsychology and the understanding and resolution of challenging behaviour in dementia.

When assessing the severity of a person's dementia, doctors and nurses test for difficulties with language, thinking, memory and orientation. When it comes to orientation we talk about a person being disoriented in time, place and person. They are asked where they are and where they live; they are asked to recognise who they are with and recall who they are talking to; and to assess time disorientation, they are asked the day, the date, the month and the year. As they struggle to remember, the impression that is given is that to lose awareness of time is similar to us losing track of the days when on holiday or puzzling over the date when there has previously been no reason to check.

While in the beginning time disorientation may be like this, it cannot remain so because changes in the parts of the brain associated with memory are so severe that the ability to retain and recall thoughts and experiences is eventually devastated. In due course it is not only the markers of time - days and dates - that are lost to memory, so is one's place in time, and it is this we need to understand.

An appreciation that time has passed relies on the capacity to store the passage of time and all that has happened. In dementia, the progressive incorrigible disabling of memory means that eventually this no longer happens. There is no recent past and only a fleeting sense of future founded on a tenuous grasp of the immediate present, which is in itself shrouded in 'not knowing'. So what does the passing of time mean to a person with dementia?

Who has not woken in the morning and on occasions during that time of transition from sleep to wakefulness not known where they are? Reassuringly, in a split second we recall and all is well. But imagine how we would feel if the penny did not drop, and despite all our efforts to remember and understand no answer was forthcoming? If we can envisage the fear and horror that would well up inside us, then welcome to the world within which a person with dementia lives. For this is their life.

Every waking moment is affected by an unremitting sense of not knowing. There is no knowledge of where one is or who others might be, and this is not solely because recent experiences can no longer be converted into memory. As established memories, both autobiographical and remote are lost, it is not only 'the new' that remains mysterious but what was once known is also rendered strange.

Yet even this understanding does not bring us close enough to the experience of dementia. To achieve true understanding we need to acknowledge a most important difference that exists between ourselves and people with dementia; a difference that is almost impossible to comprehend.

Let us return to the bedroom. If we were to be lying there, not knowing and despite all efforts to recall where we are and what is expected of us, no answer was to be found, as time passed we may gain a sense of reassurance, for nothing remarkable or threatening had transpired. Our anxieties might abate and fears might subside to be replaced by mystifying puzzlement and a determination to seek an answer. However, as dementia progresses along its unforgiving path, recent thoughts and experiences are effaced within moments. Seconds after having thought "where am I?", the query has never been raised and so the experience of questioning commences again, and then again and then again... The moment and its emotions are endlessly recycled with no prospect that the passage of time may dampen feelings of fear and alarm, for there is no sense that time has passed.

Without memory, does a person with dementia realise they have a repeated a question when they see the expression of incredulity on people's faces? When told, can they grasp the fact they must have been doing something, been somewhere, even if they cannot recollect what or where? Or does the person's precarious grasp on reality mean there is just 'now' – an immediate present with any accompanying future intentions destined to dissipate within seconds?

An experience of life that is determined by the span of memory and that which lies beyond constitutes little more than a disconnected series of ephemeral events and experiences. There is no natural flow, no underpinning narrative to provide continuity. Simply disparate events to be survived, endured – and is it beyond hope to believe also to be enjoyed? And if joy is found, it does not matter that the experience which produced laughter is not remembered, for in

no way can that diminish the happiness that was felt at the time. Conversely, that which was shameful or alarming – to have wet oneself or to be faced with somebody who screamed unintelligibly – is not to be tempered by the fact that the experience will be forgotten within seconds. If at any time the immediacy of life is unspeakably appalling then this is all life comprises.

The inevitable conclusion to be drawn is that to all intents and purposes the person has dropped out of the passage of time. All that remains is the 'here and now'. They can never again reflect on what has been enjoyed or look forward to something that has been promised, nor can they ease feelings of distress when lost and bewildered with knowledge that in the past similar experiences ended well.

Without memory, time has not passed and all that was experienced, whether it was good or ill, has never happened. For people with dementia, time passing is ultimately a concept without meaning.

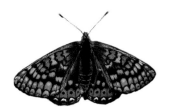

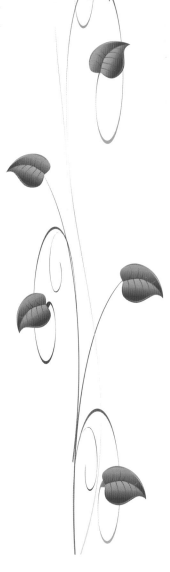

06:04

Snapshots in time

Sally Knocker

Time to look out of the window

One evening in a care home, when drawing the curtains, I stopped to notice a sunset and asked Mr Jones if he would like sit and watch it with me. I turned his wheelchair and his line of vision away from the same view he watched all day to the wider horizons of the night sky. It was a particularly beautiful sunset, taking its time to prepare for slumber and displaying its bedtime quilt of cherry and rhubarb reds, candy floss pinks and soft baby blues entwined.

It is rare for me to enjoy total silence, but for 15 minutes we sat together without words enjoying this gentle spectacle in mutual awe and reverence. It was one of those unexpected experiences rarely to be shared or savoured so intimately with another person.

Once the final bright rays had crept behind the skyscape to who-knows-where and the darker hues of night had confirmed the day's departure, we still sat for many minutes. Mr Jones finally turned to me with a smile and said in a whisper, "That's what life is all about isn't it?" He was a man with dementia for whom words and clarity of thought were hard to grasp. But in that moment we both felt it and knew.

How simple it is to turn a chair to face a window as the sun comes up or goes down, yet how easy it is to miss these natural wonders in our busy lives.

Transported in time

Mrs Hamble lived in a nursing home. She was 96 years old, very physically frail and had advanced dementia. She slept a great deal and was only able to verbalise a few repetitive words such as "Mother, mother" or "Nurse, nurse".

One afternoon I decided to take Mrs Hamble out for a walk in her wheelchair. My colleagues were a little sceptical saying that she would probably remain asleep. However, it was a crisp sunny autumn afternoon and the outside beckoned.

I went with Mrs Hamble to a small local park where leaves were falling from the tree. Sunlight was catching the beautiful array of autumn shapes and colours – oranges, yellows, browns, greens and in-betweens. Mrs Hamble was still fast asleep. I suddenly had a childish impulse (a great asset in dementia care!) to run through the leaves. So I ran kicking them in the air, lifting my arms up high to catch a falling one, enjoying the crunchy sound of contact with those at my feet and the air and sunshine on my face.

Gradually Mrs Hamble's face started to lift from her slumber as she noticed my movement and energy. She started to smile and then called out with great animation, "Run, RUN!" In that moment, the wrinkled 96-year-old face became transformed – awake, alert, alive! It was as if she had been transported in time and was six years old again in her mind and in her heart running in the leaves alongside me. Through watching another in that moment, she was able to leave behind her weak body and tired mind to find a place that was light and fun and free again.

The message behind this little story is how important it is to offer people with dementia *time to watch others* doing things so that even if they cannot physically participate, they can mentally and spiritually travel to another time and memory. Let us grasp and cherish these simple moments as elusive but lovely as the leaves themselves.

06:05

Time projections

Christian Müller-Hergl

Christian Müller-Hergl studied theology and philosophy in Bochum, Germany and Oxford. He has both worked and taught as a mental health nurse in aged care, working as home manager and matron and training in clinical supervision and organisational development. He has also taught at a college of further education for nurses. He is a Dementia Care Mapping (DCM) trainer and German strategic lead for DCM. He now works at the University of Witten/Herdecke, Institute for science in nursing, in the Dialogcenter Dementia.

Zen ideas about 'living in the moment' are in vogue lately, and I have read romantic descriptions of people with dementia living in the 'eternal present', as if they represent our better selves and a superior way of life. I think we need to be cautious about this.

People with dementia may be experiencing time in this way – sometimes described as a 'collapse of time grid' – but it is not always a happy condition. The mixture of past and present can involve – not always, but often enough – trauma-reactivation and re-traumatisation, for example during intimate care. This means that people revisit traumatic scenes and settings of their life with the same intensity of emotion as if the event had just taken place (as anyone who has cared for war veterans or abuse victims will know).

'Presence' and 'moment' in dementia are neither positive nor negative. 'Their' time is different from 'ours', but no salvation or revelation for 'us' is to be gained there. The gain for us is our own personal development and growth through living with and caring for people you only (if you try hard) half understand. The 'irreducible other' (strange, alien, frighteningly different and at the same time so similar, equal, and intimate) is the edge to sharpen awareness, imagination, and adaptive ability.

Dementia in itself has no intrinsic value, has no meaning, message or mission, personal or social. It is people with dementia and meeting them and their families that is of intrinsic value and might enable care staff to learn something about themselves – tolerance, adaptability, stress thresholds, staying power, morale and reflectivity for example.

In the real world, care staff have little chance to develop a relaxed pace and attitude. If you need to move, think and act quickly, your awareness of yourself, the other and the context is bound to deteriorate, and function will rule the day.

Recently I came down to the principle of building 'islands' of contact. I have started to support institutions to build such islands of protected time for contact between individual staff and residents, in an ocean of pressing demands and tasks to be completed. It helps to cultivate hope.

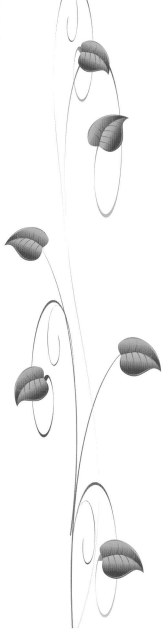

06:06

In a moment, for a moment, in the moment

Kate Allan

Kate Allan is both a clinical psychologist and a freelance consultant who works to promote understanding of the central roles of communication and creativity in supporting people who have dementia.

How often do we say to someone with dementia "I'll be with you in a moment"? It is surely a very familiar scenario: that moment may or may not come at all, may come soon or much later than hoped, and may last only a moment.

A profoundly different scenario is conjured up by changing the smallest word in the same sentence: "I'll be with you in *the* moment". What is implied by this?

For a moment, let's take a step back from the situation involving a person with dementia and think about how often we are simply 'in the moment' – experiencing something fully and immediately, without thoughts of past or present intruding, without judging or categorising? Such a state describes the practice of 'mindfulness', a discipline closely related to Buddhist forms of meditation.

But whether we have such experiences or not, what relevance could such a practice have to our daily lives, or to our work with people who have dementia?

Those who practise and teach mindfulness believe that cultivating the capacity to spend time simply being, inhabiting the present moment without criticism or comment on a daily basis is fundamental to a healthy relationship with ourselves, other people and the world around us. They believe it connects us with our own resources, alters our relationship with our thoughts and feelings, opens us up to new possibilities for action, and a new relationship with time itself (Kabat-Zinn 2004). We have evidence it is helpful for people who experience depression and anxiety, and those under stress and in pain. The ancient wisdom of

meditation has filtered through to the empirical scientists and practitioners of the 21st century.

So, returning to our scenario, imagine: you are in the moment – you see the person in front of you with new eyes, you notice new things about they way they look, sound and act. Your mind is clear and receptive, you feel open and receptive. Thoughts come and go, but you are not driven or diverted by them. The assumptions we normally bring to bear are not as compelling or controlling as usual. How much more would be possible if we could – at least some of the time – encounter persons with dementia in this way?

Perhaps this is more like the way the person with dementia experiences time too? Laura Smith, who has dementia, and helped to found the Dementia Advocacy and Support Network International, said:

Most of the time I live in the space I can see and the time called 'now'…

And drawing attention to the possibilities inherent in this state, Christine Bryden, who was diagnosed with dementia when she was in her fifties has written:

this fact that we live in the present, with a depth of spirit and some tangled emotions means you can connect with us at a deep level through touch, eye contact, smiles.

Can we learn from people with dementia to spend more of our lives in the moment?

Bryden C (2005) *Dancing with Dementia: My Story of Living Positively with Dementia.* Jessica Kingsley, London.
Smith L quoted in Bryden C (2005).
Kabat-Zinn J (2004) *Wherever you go, there you are: Mindfulness Meditation for Everyday Life.* Piatkus, London.

06:07

The fine art of living in the moment

Richard Cheston

Richard Cheston is a Consultant Clinical Psychologist working for Avon and Wiltshire Mental Health Partnership trust, and was formerly a lecturer at Bath University. He has been leading, writing about and carrying out research into short-term psychotherapy groups for people diagnosed as having a dementia for the last 15 years.

Tomorrow, and tomorrow, and tomorrow,
Creeps in this petty pace from day to day,
To the last syllable of recorded time;
And all our yesterdays have lighted fools
The way to dusty death. Out, out, brief candle!
Life's but a walking shadow, a poor player,
That struts and frets his hour upon the stage,
And then is heard no more. It is a tale
Told by an idiot, full of sound and fury,
Signifying nothing.
– William Shakespeare, *Macbeth* Act V Scene 5

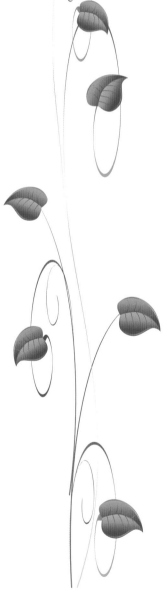

In psychotherapeutic terms, dementia can be understood as a problematic experience: that is to say, as an experience which, because of the enormity of its psychological implications, resists easy assimilation into the individual's existing self. To approach the experience of dementia fully would in existential terms be akin to looking directly into the sun: to glimpse an inexorable path of deterioration marked by the emotional dilemmas of dependence; to struggle to create some meaning from life, when the imminence of decay means that life may be rendered pointless.

For the last 15 years or so I have led a series of groups for people with dementia. The issues and problems that are raised in these groups, like the process and dynamics of being in a group, are not specifically related to the experience of dementia, even if progressive neurological deterioration is always the setting for these issues to be expressed. These concerns are essentially human concerns: they relate to the nature of being – they are existential concerns that relate to the process of living.

One thing that I have learnt is that, for many, knowing what day of the week it is, what month, or even what season or year it is, is just not that important any more. Now, we could take a position that this indifference is itself a sign of neurological impairment, perhaps involving the frontal lobes that are responsible for executive functioning. But often these people that I work with who do not know what month or season or year it is, and do not especially care that they do not know, do care about other things. Indeed, they often care very passionately about these other things. They may care, for instance, that they stay in their homes and do not go into nursing care. They may care when others call them 'gaga' or suggest that there is something seriously wrong with them. Their neurological impairment, then, does not extend to a global indifference – rather the carelessness is a very particular form of indifference. Asked to explain their indifference, they may comment to the effect that these things are not important, or that if they really needed to know, then they could ask someone else who did know.

We cannot begin to explore these experiences without the context of time – just as distance lends enchantment, so time provides a perspective on one's life. Confronted by the overwhelming loss of perspective – of the ruins of an imagined future, and of an immediate past that is shrunken and violated, so the temptation for the person with dementia is to live within the moment. This moment, this here-and-now becomes all; and with the loss of time, ie the loss of perspective, so too a sense of responsibility goes. The person with dementia may focus and stay within the here-and-now. This is an adaptive response: it doesn't matter what the date is, what the year or month of the year is, so long as you exist in the moment – then all can feel well. You are surviving. Time becomes a commodity that you cannot afford – it is jettisoned as irrelevant and as unimportant. Only from the outside, for those of us who are concerned with the importance of an orientation in person, time and place, does a concern with time seem vital.

To lose one's focus on the moment is to risk becoming aware of time's winged chariot, hurrying near. Not being aware of time is one way of loosening the grip of an existential threat caused by cognitive deterioration, increasing dependence and the imminence of death. This is not to say that people don't know what day it is. Rather it is to acknowledge that they don't care to try to know.

In a number of different forms of psychotherapy in recent years, it has grown popular to encourage one's clients to learn techniques of 'mindfulness'. These ideas have a long history in many different cultures, including being drawn from practices of meditation and Buddhist teachings. The essential idea is that individuals need to live in the moment – a feature of depression or anxiety is the difficulty to stay grounded in what is going on around oneself. Instead the mind is crowded with worried thoughts and ruminations about what ought to be, about the imagined future and the troubled past. The solution to anxiety or depression that comes from a too close engagement with life's uncertainties, and with one's human frailties, then, is to help the person to be invested in the moment that is lived – in the here-and-now.

Let us imagine for a moment ourselves that we are so cursed with dementia that we struggle to recognise who we are, or where we exist, to put names to the faces of our companions, or even to recognise that their faces are familiar. We might be tempted to remove our thinking, to place ourselves within the moment, to leave responsibility to those around us who would pick it up. We might want to cultivate this fine art of living in the moment – to be simply in the here-and-now, and to exist in our memories of the there-and-then. This would be preferable, I should imagine, to facing the sun and risk glimpsing between our fingers, pressed across our eyes to protect us from its glare, the terror of an imagined future.

To those around us we might seem to have become deadened and impaired – our focus on the here-and-now might seem to them to be another sign that we had lost our mind to deterioration. This comforting myth of deterioration would be preferable for them, perhaps, to glimpsing their own imagined future, when they too might need to grasp this existential crisis for themselves.

06:08

A moment in time

Jenny La Fontaine

Jenny La Fontaine is a Research Officer at the Oxford Institute of Ageing and an Admiral Nurse with Worcestershire Mental Health Partnership Trust and for dementia. She has worked with people affected by dementia and their families for most of her 30-year career as a nurse. She continues to practise with families affected by dementia, and develop the practice of others. Her current research study involves exploring how the relationship between grandparents and their younger grandchildren is affected by dementia.

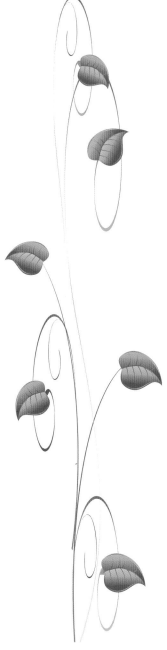

A moment in time, sharing together
A walk in a park, communicating but not
  referring to the difficulties that one has
A shared sight of a rare bird, a smile,
Both not knowing the name but knowing
  the sight
Togetherness, sharing a connection without
  words

A moment in time, being together
A walk around a nature centre
The object of our shared time, a beautiful
  snowy owl with its back to us
A whistle from one of us, causes it to turn
  its head
Laughter ensued, delight at the reaction,
  and delight at the connection
Words unnecessary,
A shared moment of time, joy and
  togetherness

A moment in time, the end is coming
Standing in a corridor
I don't understand, trying to make sense
  of this knot
One patiently trying to undo the knot while
  the other stands
Trust for a moment in time

A moment in time,
Standing in a corridor
Lost and alone, no one can hear me
You are here,
The sound of your voice and the touch of
  your hand
No longer lost for that moment in time,
I am alive for that moment in time

A moment in time
I hear of your death
An opportunity to reflect upon
A memory of a person who shared of
  themself
Who taught me empathy and compassion
And who enabled me to value those
  moments in time

06:09

A transcendent doorway to 'soul moments'

Judith Maizels

Judith Maizels was born in London in 1948. She studied earth sciences, enjoying an academic career at Aberdeen University. She became ill with ME, which eventually forced her to take early retirement, after which she became an intuitive artist, setting up and running an arts charity. Once she was well again, she combined her creative work with being a part-time carer for her parents, both of whom developed dementia, and is currently writing a self-help book on recovery from chronic illness.

Both my parents suffered from dementia – my dad had vascular dementia, and certainly did suffer (with torment and frightening delusions). He died over two years ago. My mum has Alzheimer's and went into a care home 18 months ago. I have documented much of my experience over these years, not with the original intention of publishing but to help me cope with and process events and experiences of such huge emotional intensity. Time has proved both an enemy and a friend: an enemy in that it took my dad from me too soon, but a friend in relieving him from his torment. A friend too in that my mother's Alzheimer's has taken her to a new world so slowly, over nearly a whole decade, that I have found myself somehow adjusting to the different parts of herself which have emerged with each passing year – from her initial frightened, insecure self; to her tormented, angry, demanding self, desperate to 'go home'; to the calm, deeply contented, kindly soul who now greets me on my arrival at the care home.

The thought of my mum moving into a home was originally anathema to me; I resisted any suggestion of such a thing from carers and family. But eventually I realised that my mum herself wanted this when I discovered she preferred to stay at her day centre rather than go home (she had a live-in carer).

While it was traumatic for me to see my mum arriving in a place full of frightening (for me) strangers with dementia, she settled in straight away. After several years of demanding to go home every single day, since moving she has not once mentioned 'going home' – she *is* at home and the last year (her 89th) has been one of the happiest of her life.

But for me, it took about six months to come to terms with her move – and much to my astonishment and with much humility, I now realise that this last year has been one of the most moving, tender, enlightening and precious years of my own life. The lessons are many, and of these the most profound have been learning to cherish the moment; to be open to, accepting of, and celebrating whatever awaits me on each visit; to cherish my relationship with my mother, now not 'reduced to', but 'enriched to', its very essence: love. Mother, daughter, sister, friend, the name doesn't matter anymore. And I have felt humbled and touched to discover the sweet essence that lies in the heart of so many of her companions – now innocents, vulnerable and often tormented. Similarly, I have witnessed many tender encounters between the residents and the care staff, and built relationships which have helped to support me too.

This has indeed been a journey of transformation for me. At first I used to call my journey in the lift up to the 'Reminiscence Community' as taking me 'halfway to Hell', but now I feel it is really 'halfway to Heaven'. As I travel upwards in the lift I silently pray for light, love and healing for all. When the door opens, I take a deep breath, and step forward through a doorway into a different world. Here time itself takes on a different dimension. Time does not pass faster or more slowly than in the outer world; instead, it takes on a transcendent quality. My experience of time is transformed, reflecting the fact that the emotional intensity of each moment seems to become vividly heightened.

For example, by the time the door opens, I have prepared myself to be open, accepting, receptive and loving, with whatever comes. My attention becomes focused on whatever awaits me, as I try to engage with my mother, and other residents, in whatever place they are at that very moment. I find myself in a state of heightened awareness, all my senses becoming more alive - reaching out, smiling, touching, talking, laughing, listening, just being fully present with each person and how they are. I try to let go of my own fears and anxieties, of my own ego; not rushing or having any expectations, not watching the clock. These qualities remind me of a meditation, when we focus our attention on our breath. We know that meditation of this kind can bring neurological and physiological benefits associated with being fully present in the moment. And indeed, sharing this time together often fills me with a spiritual joy, forming 'soul moments' on my own journey. The community, both residents and care staff, have allowed me to step inside that magic doorway, to reveal what is most important in this life: unconditional love.

Of course, each visit is a powerful mix of joy, pain and grief, but joy is usually the victor - because love is so strong and reaches out to touch so many souls, living in that world apart, as they travel together on their solitary timeless journey. I am trying to journey alongside, so that each step feels less solitary, and each soul more loved; both theirs and my own. For this powerful new experience of time, I am deeply grateful to all those courageous and inspiring travellers ahead of me on the road.

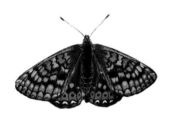

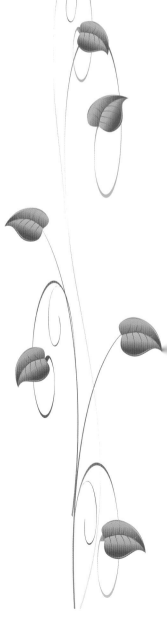

06:10

Don't forget today

Dave Anderson

Dr Dave Anderson is Consultant and Honorary Senior Lecturer in Old Age Psychiatry, and Chair of the Faculty of Old Age Psychiatry, Royal College of Psychiatrists.

Time defines us. I am unique because I occupy a time-space location that nobody can share. Whatever else that I am, that makes me unique.

Am I the same person I was yesterday? Ten or 50 years ago? I think not. I certainly don't recognise that person in the photographs. Nor do I understand some of the things that person did. I have changed but at every moment I was unique by occupying that time-space location. This would be the same if I had dementia.

The importance of time is demonstrated by the number of phrases we use involving the word. Time and tide, in the nick of time, at the best of times, the passage of time, having had one's time, take one's time, the time of life.

My preference is: there's no time like the present. The future is imponderable and impossible to predict. The past is useful for learning (though only in the present) and pleasant for reminiscence, though we remember it more as we wish than as it was. The now is all we have. If every now moment is fulfilling, life is good.

The person with dementia is exactly the same as all of us in relation to time. Though their connection between time past and time present is different, they are unique, changing and living in the present.

Facing sudden illness is frightening but living with chronic illness, particularly progressive disabling illness, is hard. In the early stages of this condition, early detection enables the person with dementia to be included, informed and in control. The opportunity to plan some things for the future is a benefit but the unpredictable nature of the passage of time means these things may never happen or be needed. Our worst fears may never happen and anticipating them wouldn't make them any less awful. And the person I worry about may no longer be here.

Yet, so often, the present of people with dementia and their families is dominated by worry of the future. What can we expect? How long will someone live? What is going to happen? What is my risk of getting this? Will he become aggressive? What sort of care home will she need? She won't be able to live at home then? Will he need to be sedated? How will we manage if he starts wandering? What shall we do if she can't look after herself? What do we do if he won't take his medication? Or people are overwhelmed by sadness of loss because they can only think about the past.

As memory fails, nobody lives more in the present than a person with dementia. Their understanding of the present may be mistaken but when things are forgotten within minutes, life is truly in the instant. At every moment that person is thinking, deciding, acting in the instant. If we understand their sense of the present we can understand them.

The problems that arise from dementia arise in the present and we need to manage them in the present, not the past or the future. If we can do that today and every day, life is fulfilling and successful.

Accept me as I am now. Understand me today not as I was yesterday or how I may be tomorrow. If you can, you might prescribe me fewer drugs, you might enforce fewer rules that don't make sense to me, you might stop expecting me to be someone I used to be. I'm sorry I can't remember you but if you know me could you accept me as I am now? Every day I'm me but every day is different and this is the me today. Thank you for loving all of the 'me's of the past but if that's all you see then you won't be able to love the me of today. Make the best of every present moment for, though time is infinite, a human life is not.

If we spend today only thinking of tomorrow or yesterday, we will miss today, forget to appreciate and enjoy the experience of the relationship with that person.

In King John, Shakespeare called time "that bald sexton" represented with a lock of hair on his forehead but none on the rest of his head, showing that time past cannot be used but time present may be seized by the forelock. Live with people today, enjoy them today, laugh with them today, help them today, for today is all we have.

As the Zen writer Daniel Levin writes, "This moment is the only thing that's real. Worrying about the future and lamenting the past only crowds out the beauty of what is happening now."

When we think about the person with dementia let us not forget today. If we forget today then all we have has gone.

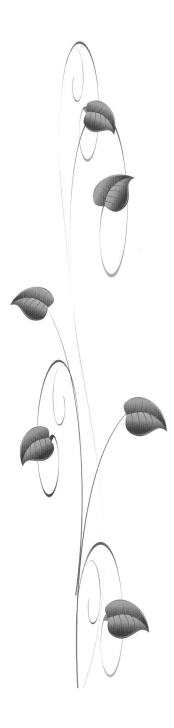

A poor life this if, full of care,
We have no time to stand and stare.
WH Davies
From 'Leisure'

06:11

Taking time in the present

Faith Gibson

Faith Gibson is an emeritus professor of social work from the University of Ulster. She has a long-standing interest in reminiscence work and especially in encouraging people with dementia to recall memories as a means for promoting communication and enriching relationships in the present.

While the past is a rich resource for many people who have dementia it is also essential for carers of all kinds to be alert to seizing every opportunity, even if fleeting, for engaging with people in the present. Although memories of the past are a rewarding reservoir on which to draw, and without a sense of time past people may feel adrift in time present, the present is all that any of us can actually know. While we may be able to recall the past and imagine a future, we cannot know either in the way we experience the present. While people with dementia can often recall the more distant past, even if the recent past eludes them, they may well have difficulty in imagining the future.

In so many ways people with dementia are expert existentialists – they live from moment to moment so that the quality of the present becomes all important. With probably impaired ability to formulate future plans, envision the future, let alone recall on demand the immediate past or, eventually, the more distant past too, they are compelled to live in the moment. Angela Tilbey, a priest and broadcaster captured this idea when recently referring to a person with dementia who talked about "the sacrament of the present moment".

Experience suggests that while the past indeed may be in our hearts and those of people experiencing dementia, it is the present that provides opportunities for pleasure and reassurance. The present may equally of course be a source of distress, discomfort and anxiety. The challenge for carers is to make the present as stress free, enjoyable and companionable as possible despite the many life reducing challenges dementia presents. These challenges may include current living arrangements and environmental limitations, encroaching social isolation, strained or lost relationships, curtailed liberty and restricted choices along with unreliable and uncontrollable cognitive malfunctioning. The onus must be on carers to lessen the impact of disturbance in people's perception of time and to share in the pleasure of the present moment, no matter how brief or transitory such encounters may be.

Thus care environments, while containing reminders of time and place which some people may find helpful, must also provide indispensable reassuring warm companionship. This is the essential bulwark that may enable the present not only to be endured but also to be enjoyed. Members of care staff need their managers to reorder work priorities. They need to be assisted to set aside incessant busyness, to learn to value brief encounters as well as longer periods of conversation, too often undervalued or dismissed as 'just chatting'. And all of us must learn how to join the time frame or step into the world as perceived by people with dementia, to be still, to appreciate how each person situates themselves in time and place and not insist that they join our world or feel demeaned and impoverished as they struggle to retain a tenuous hold upon the brittle thread of the present.

06:12

Time in reverse

Roxann Johnson

Roxann Johnson is a third year PhD student in the Department of Applied Social Science at the University of Stirling in Scotland. Her current research interests are dementia and front-line care workers. She is conducting cross-national comparison of training for front-line care workers in care homes in Canada, Scotland and the United States.

The concept of time can be as elusive as the various forms of dementia. For people with dementia, time metaphorically speaks volumes. To look at time from another perspective, for an insightful view, consider time in reverse, literally and figuratively. Time spelled backwards is emit, which means "to give utterance or voice to". To honour the concept of time for people with dementia we must allow them the opportunity to emit their messages. It could be with words, gestures or simply an expression.

In our youth, time lingered for what felt like an eternity. As the years go by our memories, life and time seem to fly by. My dear mother-in-law once said, "Time stands still for a moment as my life races through my mind in fast forward and in the blink of an eye I'm in the slow lane searching for words to express my thoughts, hoping that someone will be there… to listen." When I looked into her eyes our gaze locked, igniting a spark that emitted a beautiful contented smile. I knew that for that instant we were there together, only if it was for just a moment, we shared that moment in time. For that day my purpose was to be there and allow her the time and opportunity to emit her message and to smile and say, "Oh yes… I know you."

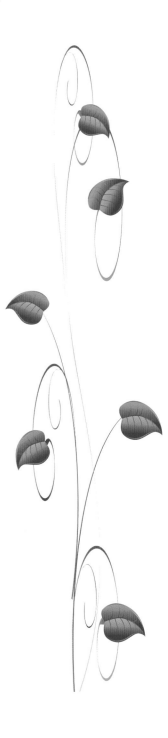

Paradox

Murna Downs

Murna Downs is Chair in Dementia Studies and Head of the Bradford Dementia Group at Bradford University. Her research interests focus on quality of life and quality of care for people with dementia and their families.

time
slips
slides
swirls
curls
bringing us
to places forgotten
to a present that is the past
to the moment that is all there is

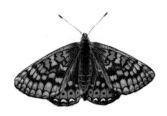

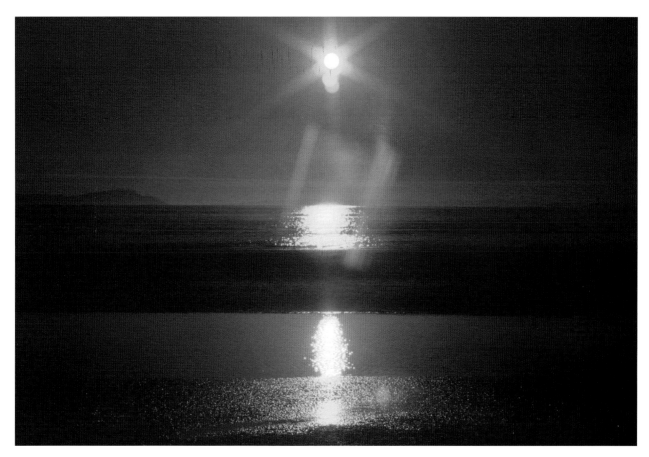

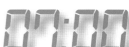

Night time

07:01

Time during night shift

Fiona Kelly

Fiona Kelly is a practising nurse and has worked with people with dementia for over 15 years. She completed her doctorate in 2007 and is currently a lecturer in dementia studies at the Dementia Services Development Centre at the University of Stirling. She has a strong commitment to improving practice in the support and care of people with dementia, in particular those who live in long-term care.

I am in the privileged position of having two jobs in the dementia field. The first is working with a great team of people in the Dementia Services Development Centre, at the University of Stirling, where I lecture in dementia studies, have access to current thinking in dementia care and regularly meet and share ideas with extraordinary and passionate people.

My other job is nursing people with dementia in a little nursing home close to where I live. This is home to 13 people with dementia – 13 amazing, loving, creative and unique people who have taught me about humanity, love, humour, patience and the value of time. My preferred shift is a night shift, because of the qualitatively different use of time and passing of time that I experience. Working on a night shift has its own momentum, its own pace which is not governed by pressures to achieve tasks, but which drifts and flows with a slowness that allows for a different experience of caring. On night shift, in this special little home, there is an abundance of time which makes working during these sleeping hours a uniquely special and rewarding experience.

On my shift, there is:

time to really listen
time to sit in companionship
time to chat and share stories
time to watch the sunset and marvel at the moon
time to bring in the washing and smell the sweetness of the fading day
time to spend holding the hand of someone who is dying
time to accompany them along their final journey
time to sing and sometimes to dance
time to hug and to be hugged
time for humour and rhymes
time to spend time
time for quietness
time to attend
time to reflect
time to be.

This is the privilege of working the night shift.

07:02

Night time

Diana Kerr

Diana Kerr is a research fellow at the University of Edinburgh. Her area of research is predominantly in the field of learning disability and dementia. She has, however, just completed research concerned with 'Supporting older people in care homes at night'. Diana is an advisor to service providers and planners and a trainer to health and social work staff on dementia.

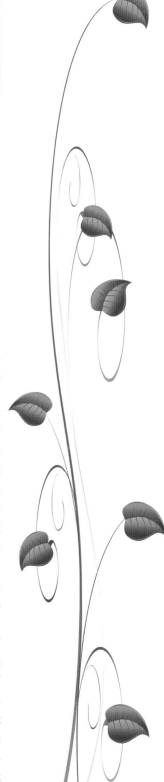

Night time and day time are different, 'as different as day and night'. Night time, the hours between 10pm and 6am, is the time when the dark descends, when the world is shut away, and when 'our nightly appointment with death' becomes the time when fears and worries take hold. The night hours seem longer than the day hours. The night time, which can hold us in slumber and peace can also be the time of fear and turmoil as we endure the dark watches of the night. How often do we wake in the morning to find the fears of the night to be gone or at least diminished?

In the still of the night, time changes, it dislocates, it fools and extends. The anchors and cues of the day time are gone and the night time ticks slowly

For people with dementia this stillness and emptiness can be particularly frightening and disorientating. Dementia takes people back in time. They need cues and help to orientate. Alone, at night, there are none. The person with dementia is trapped in the past, unable to understand the present. The damage to the circadian rhythm, the mechanism that regulates our body clock, telling us the difference between day time and night time, means that people with dementia will often misinterpret or mistrust such night time cues as do exist. People will often assume that if they wake it is morning and time for the tasks of the new day rather than the task of the night time, to sleep.

He wakes to find the bed
Half empty. She has gone

Past midnight, in her nightgown,
Four streets and eighteen years astray.

A policeman brings her home.
He leads her back to bed.

He holds her, sobbing till she sleeps
(Clancy 2000)

The conviction that the night has passed can be so strong that any cues that do exist are often ignored.

A man with dementia always got up at 7am to go to work. Because of the effect of the dementia when he woke at 3am he assumed it really must be seven. Undaunted by the fact that the clock showed 3am, he decided that the timepiece was wrong and he was right. He then changed the hands, and the time, to 7am. Perhaps he just wanted the night to end.

A good way to deal with the fears of the night time might be to speed it up and get to the daytime as quickly as possible!

Generally, despite the specific needs of people with dementia, services still continue to provide night time care and support as if the night time was a time when people are continually asleep, are not distressed and not in need of reassurance. The consequence is that night staff ratios in care homes are inappropriately lower than for the day time, night staff are less well trained in the night time needs of people with dementia and night time environments are not designed to compensate for the disabilities of the condition (Kerr *et al* 2008).

The night time is hidden and often under-supervised, under-inspected and under-resourced. This is precisely because it *is* the night time, the time when the 'ordinary' world sleeps.

Night time for people with dementia needs to be what it is for the rest of us: a time for peace, calm, reflection, restoration and preparation. Night time for people with dementia must be brought into the light, better understood, properly resourced, and properly supported. This will only happen when the time at night is seen as an integral and significant part of the whole 24 hours of the day.

Clancy J (2000) *Ordinary Time*. Gomer, Ceredigion.
Kerr D, Wilkinson H, Cunningham C (2008) *Supporting People in Care Homes at Night*. Joseph Rowntree Foundation. York.

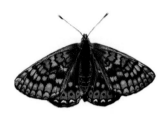

07:03

'Have a good night!'
'We will do our best to respect your rhythm and your customs'

Marie-Jo Guisset-Martinez & Marion Villez

Marie-Jo Guisset-Martinez and Marion Villez work for the Fondation Méderic Alzheimer which exists to build up innovative practice and to promote, support and evaluate new initiatives in dementia care in France. It also undertakes research. Marie-Jo, a social worker, is the programme manager and she also coordinates two European networks. Marion is the programme's assistant and she is undertaking a PhD in sociology. They have both written numerous publications about dementia care.

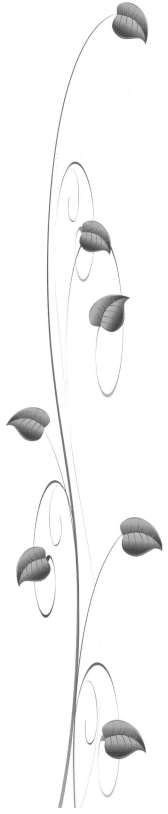

Be it at home or in an institution, the night is a period during which people with dementia and their carers experience exceptionally difficult situations which are, paradoxically, hardly spoken about… unknown times, feared times.

At home, at the end of the afternoon, the person with dementia can feel anxiety, sleep a little, and walk from room to room looking for the toilet without finding it. The carer can be in permanent fear of an accident. When the person with dementia lives alone the relatives are anxious about real or imaginary risks and dangers, which can make the situation unacceptable in the long run.

In France, for some years, a few night care support programmes such as temporary/ sequential facilities or mobile night services have been provided. (Guisset-Martinez 2007). The objective of the night care facility is to give a break once or twice a week to the spouse or child who sleeps in the vicinity of the person whose sleeping rhythms are not easily manageable. In Normandy-Montain the local geriatric hospital has a sequential residential care programme offering a range of possibilities from day care to short-term breaks, allowing a flexible response to the needs of people with dementia and their families. The programme incorporates consistent elements to reassure and comfort the person making the trip from home to hospital. For instance, the same driver comes to fetch the person at home in the late afternoon and brings them back the next morning after breakfast.

Mobile night care visits can be scheduled for a specific purpose or through a subscription, or as an emergency. Requests for assistance include help to go to sleep, to get up, for basic hygiene during the night or regular visits to check all is well. Nachtzorg in Antwerp, Belgium, for example, was founded in 2004 to allow the person with dementia to live for as long as possible in good circumstances, and to support and relieve carers. Nachtzorg brings support, comfort and care between 9.30pm and 6.30am to 25 people. The recent French dementia plan (2008) underlines the necessity of developing more night facilities.

In France and in many other countries, in spite of a few existing services, the problems encountered at night by carers can be the tipping point behind the family's decision to opt for the solution of permanent residential care. But in care homes too the night is often far from being a quiet, restful time for staff and residents. Some people with dementia have problems which cause discomfort to them as well as roommates and neighbours. Some people do not sleep. They walk around and cause disruption by repeated and insistent attempts to open all closed doors and go into other people's rooms. Night is the time for insomnia in people who have not had much activity during the day and have perhaps dozed as a result of boredom, fatigue or drug treatments.

Observing, listening and trying to understand and help people through the night is a challenge. Several strategies are used by care teams. Human presence is an undeniable factor of reassurance. Some people are woken by hunger. In many facilities the rather light evening meal is served quite early. A resident with communication problems may not be able to express hunger. It is a good idea to offer small snacks spontaneously, to calm both anxiety and hunger, as well as to create an opportunity for contact with staff on night duty.

Some people are afraid of the dark, so a light can be left on in the room. Lights left on in the lounge help bring together people looking for company. Mattresses on the floor permit a person, soothed by human presence, to fall asleep once calmed.

Close attention allowed the staff of La Salette nursing home near Lyon, in France, to understand the behaviour of certain people who were tired and anxious during the day but very active at night. Their project 'To each his life, to each his night' came out of a brainstorming involving day and night care teams. Together, which is quite exceptional, they were able to understand, for instance, why a former baker and a former nurse did not sleep much during the night. The 'night programme' was then designed in individually tailored plans: making cakes for the retired baker, watching movies for a sophisticated cinema fan. End result – fewer night anxieties and lower doses of sleeping pills, livelier days and calmer nights.

It can help for night staff (as in Carpe Diem, Quebec, Canada) to wear pyjamas or informal clothes, so that when a person with dementia walks around it is easier to explain that it is night time and to invite them to go back to bed.

Preparing for a good night can be helpful. A good night's sleep incorporates several dimensions and preparation can take place throughout the day. First of all, a full day will generate a need for rest. Not preventing people from walking during the day, or even better suggesting an interesting walk, produces a natural, healthy fatigue and may lead to the need for rest.

For night staff, the lack of interest in their challenges can lead to a feeling of isolation. This neglect of night-time means that policy puts focus only on safety. But we believe that night time should be seen as a time for person-centred, relational support to people with dementia in the same way that this is expected during the day. As we can see, there is still a lot to do to change many institutional rules and routines. Challenges for professionals are to be able to work with an open mind and with creativity. With their empirical approach, some of the pioneers whose projects we have presented above have initiated changes which were later validated by the authorities and by legislation, in France at least.

Guisset-Martinez MJ (2007) *Care and support for people with dementia: a new deal. Reference points for professional practices.* Fondation Mederic Alzheimer, Paris.
French Dementia Plan (2008) *Alzheimer et maladies apparentees 2008-2012.* www.sante.gouv.fr/htm/dossiers/alzheimer/plam.

07:04

Night time at home

Fiona Taylor

Fiona Taylor is currently a service manager in the older adults team in North Lanarkshire Council. She is responsible for the development and integration of services. Although the majority of her remit is focused on the development of services for older adults she also oversees the continued development of the council's assistive technology service, which is available to anyone who needs it and covers all care groups.

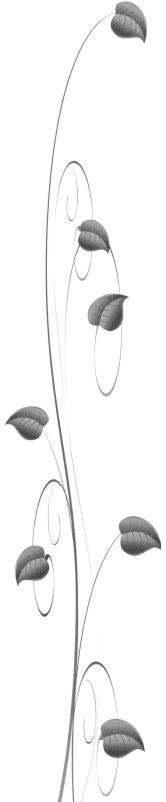

Ms Brown was first referred to the social work department by her GP who asked for a 'nursing home assessment'. The social worker who was allocated the case felt that this would be a bit hasty, and that they could provide a range of services that could support Ms Brown to live in her own home for some time yet. The initial assessment did however highlight a few significant risks in Ms Brown's lifestyle.

Ms Brown was 80 years of age and lived alone in the main street of a small town in Scotland. As she was an only child who had never married she had no immediate relatives and although she had a few neighbours who helped out now and again, these too were becoming frailer and less able.

Ms Brown had arthritis in her hands which made many ordinary living tasks very difficult and sometimes painful for her. She was also a bit forgetful, but liked to be independent and was not prepared to be told what to do or when to do it.

Ms Brown had worked as a nurse all her life and particularly enjoyed working nights. She always liked the quietness of night time and stated she still found great pleasure in looking out of her window at night at the various constellations. Sometimes she even sat in the garden and enjoyed the view on cold winter nights along with a "wee whisky".

As she had worked shifts all her life she had what some people would consider to be an erratic sleep pattern and she ate and slept at odd times throughout the day and night. Sometimes she decided not to get dressed and to have a lazy day in her pyjamas. And at other times she had a burst of energy and decided to clear out all her drawers and cupboards during the night.

Her memory loss was having some impact on her life and with growing regularity she forgot to take her medication, and then took a few together to make up for the missed ones. She was not quite sure how often she ate, but assured the worker she was well fed and that there was always plenty of chocolate in case she felt hungry. Her neighbours were worried about her being out at night and spoke of the many days when she did not get dressed. The local greengrocer supplied her with her weekly shopping and she always had the payment sitting ready for him. As the post office was only a few doors away she continued to collect her own pension, but when the pavements were icy the owner phoned her and arranged for someone to pop along with it for her.

Provision of services

A home support service was arranged to assist Ms Brown with washing, dressing, food preparation and getting ready for bed each night. Visits were arranged three times each day, seven days a week. As an extra precaution the overnight visiting service was alerted and asked to call in if there were lights on in the house, and a key safe was fitted to allow the staff easy access.

However, within the first few weeks it became increasingly obvious that the care package was not working. Although there were times when Ms Brown was glad of the help around the house during the day, there were other times when she became quite aggressive towards the night support staff and either refused to co-operate or else she put them out of her house. As tensions rose she became quite agitated and was regularly found knocking on the doors of neighbours to complain about intruders in her home at all hours of the night.

A case conference was arranged and at that point in time it seemed that the most obvious outcome would be an admission into care. However, during the case discussion one of the student social workers who were in attendance suggested that perhaps assistive technology could be tried to support Ms Brown, as a last resort before arranging an admission to a care home.

New care package

A selection of passive infra red beams (PIRs) was fitted in the house; these were linked to the local call centre but set with time delay switches. These would inform overnight visiting staff when Ms Brown was actually up during the night, therefore preventing them popping in when she was sleeping and ensuring she had the opportunity to open the door to them if she wished.

A PIR reminder light was fitted to her front door. The home support worker activated this when she left in the evening and this reminded Ms Brown not to go out of the front door, as it was not safe. This was deactivated by the support staff in the morning as the risks were considerably less during the day and the assessor did not want to prevent her from going out and chatting to neighbours and friends in the local community. Her back door was fitted with a time delay door contact. This meant that if Ms Brown chose to go out at night to sit in her back garden, she could do so, and only if she had not come back in within the hour would the overnight staff be alerted.

As Ms Brown was often quite active during the night clearing out cupboards and tidying up when she felt energetic, the overnight visiting service was asked not to interrupt this routine, but to take this opportunity to offer tea and a light snack if they were invited in. This would make up for any meals she would decline the following day when she was tired.

The home support staff that supported Ms Brown during the day and night were provided with digital pens (see footnote) – this meant that they could send each other messages to say what she had eaten, whether she had slept and when she was most likely to need support again. In this way the workers could fit in with what suited her best rather than calling in when she had just gone to sleep or making her breakfast shortly after she had just had a snack from the overnight service.

Change of support plan

When the technology was originally installed the technicians put in place an automatic lighting system. This meant that when Ms Brown arose in the dark, lights were activated that ensured she could find her way to the toilet safely; these would turn themselves off when she was back in bed. However, these were quickly removed as staff soon discovered that Ms Brown became very agitated and could not return to bed when the lights were still on. She was worried not only about her electric bills but because she wondered who had put the lights on and thought there was someone in her house.

Eventually staff found that a touch lamp would provide sufficient lighting to allow her to go to the toilet, without having to fiddle with a small switch, and she could easily switch this off herself on her return to bed.

Ms Brown continues to enjoy living in her own home with her own routine, and is supported by staff when she needs it.

Digital pens – these are electronic pens that have a small camera inserted just beside the nib. When someone writes a note or draws a diagram, this is photographed and sent to a pre-programmed mobile phone number. In this case study the digital pen was left in the person's home beside their communication pager and the four home support staff who regularly provided a service to Ms Brown were given mobile phones to aid their communication.

07:05

Grey or gray?

Raymond Tallis

Raymond Tallis is Emeritus Professor of Geriatric Medicine at the University of Manchester, a philosopher, poet and novelist. His recent books include *The Enduring Significance of Parmenides: Unthinkable Thought* (Continuum, 2007), *The Kingdom of Infinite Space. A Fantastical Journey Around Your Head* (Atlantic, 2008), *Hunger* (Acumen, 2008) and *Michelangelo's Finger: An Investigation of Pointing* (Atlantic, 2010). He is currently writing *De Luce: An Inquiry into Human Possibility* which has been in progress for 25 years but is due to be delivered to Atlantic in 2010.

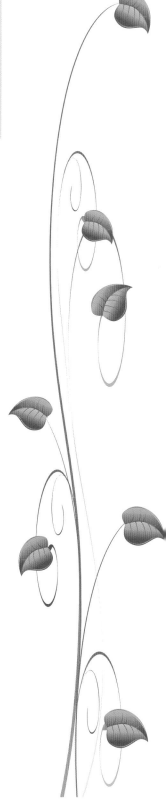

The poplars by the silvered railway tracks
are shimmerless this marbled moonlit hour.
Autumn pruned those vocal leaves, butterflies
that fretted open-windowed nights
and goosed the pools of shallow, sweaty sleep.

Only bits of ghosts trouble Auntie's house –
dream-moths zigging and zagging from
the ruined brocade and broken springs of
   time –
set free by the permissiveness of sleep.
And the soliloquies of the fridge,
and the monosyllables of the dripping tap
and the gas fire's unremitting sigh,
until the time-tabled catastrophe of the late,
   late train –
so late, it's almost early – violates
stillness with murderous haste.
Unoccupied, a gut empty of all but light,
its pointless hurry mocks the seriousness
   of rush.

Auntie wakes into grammarless wondering,
   wanders
the boscage flanking disused lanes of
   thought,
blinks at dunnocks of memory and moves
at the behest of time-bleached wants and old
   concerns,
mice under a pile of rags,
leftovers from days as scalar as cut grass.

Bent on being bent on being,
purposed by the illusion of purpose
she zimmers her ninety years to the
   open door.
Night-gowned in the street,
brailles past monadic streetlamps towards
imaginary shopping hours in memory stores
deregulated as her mind.

Like me, purposive without final purpose;
unsure, like me, which vowel is right
or where to find the final sense of things.

ROMANCE

I fell in love.
All on me own.
And he fell in love with me.
I didn't believe him.
He wouldn't tell me his name.
He says "I'll come and
I'll see you settled down."
And now he's sleeping with me.
But They've found out.

There's a shelf above the wardrobe
where I keep his pyjamas.
Oh, I'm alright with him,
In fact he's just my type.
The other night I put his pyjamas
in a drawer. I was asleep
when he came in. He didn't know
what to do. "Well why didn't you
climb in naked?" I asked him after.
Don't ask me where he works.
Making bodies. Car engines, you know?

First time I've slept
with anybody since
me husband died.
He makes me happy.
Not right happy, but
happy enough. Well, you know
what fellas are like, though?

John Killick
John Killick wrote down the words of a person with dementia in a care home to make this poem.
He then shared it back with her and obtained her approval to publish.
It comes from the collection *Dementia Diary*
(Hawker Publications 2008)

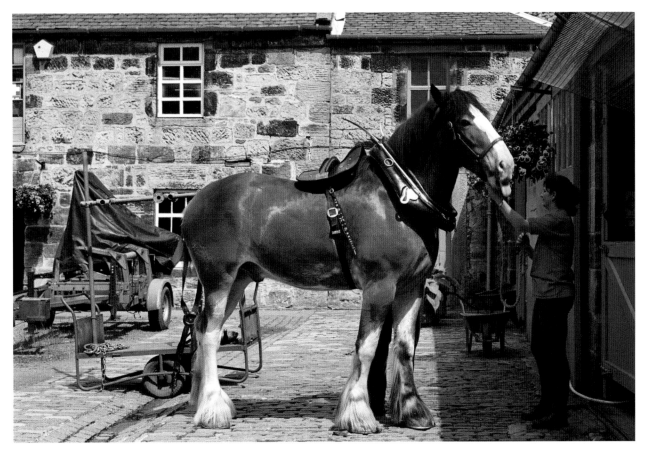

08:00

Past times

08:01

It was another country

Margaret-Anne Tibbs

Margaret Anne Tibbs is a social worker. She worked for 10 years with people living with dementia for Bedfordshire Social Services Department. For the past decade she has been a trainer/consultant in person-centred dementia care. She has been involved for many years with the Alzheimer's Society and she is the author of two social work text books on dementia, published in 2001 and 2006.

We first met over 50 years ago, but then I was a student and you and your husband, Michael, were friends of my parents. Time is strange. How I am only a couple of steps behind you on the moving escalator.

So much we have in common. Our faith, our shared history as whites in South Africa who were part of the anti-apartheid struggle. And, most significantly, you were there when my brother was drowned at Mazeppa Bay. Was it his fault, Michael asked? That my parents chose to take us to that hotel on the Wild Coast, which you loved so much? A dangerous coast and a hotel with no life saving equipment. No lifeguard – not even a life belt. He has wondered that for 49 years.

It is so long ago and yet it is no time at all. We were changed. South Africa has changed too – beyond all our wildest dreams; apartheid dismantled without bloodshed. Something we never dared to expect.

We left. You came back here to Johannesburg: to Alexandra Township to continue the apparently hopeless fight against social ills spawned by apartheid. You shared your home near Alex with Gogo and the children. Your beautiful adopted black daughter was shot dead by her partner and it broke your hearts. But you stayed until Parkinson's meant they could no longer care for you at home. When you left you made your house over to them.

I often think about how our world disappeared completely. It lives now only in the memories of its citizens. It is not like that in England, where there is unbroken continuity with the past. South Africa always had many worlds. Ours was populated by people of different races, drawn together illegally by their commitment to political change.

Some of the old worlds survive. In Pretoria we found shopping malls and suburbs still largely inhabited by whites, just about hanging on to the past. But it is different. In the old days, people's houses were not surrounded by security fences, with signs advertising armed response teams promising to come if the alarm goes, ready to shoot on sight.

In the old days the white suburbs were peaceful. It was in town that you saw the armed police. Resentment, hatred and fear which you could almost taste, held in check by omnipresent state power. Most whites never visited townships where blacks lived. But you came back to Alex. You are amazing.

One new world is that of blacks with money: also living behind security fences. The South Africa of poor blacks is familiar. In the squatter camps, the young men trying to sell you things at the traffic lights. The soaring crime rate. The horrifying statistics of multiple deprivation.

The citizens of our South Africa came from all races, Christian and Communist and all stations in between. Did the danger deepen our friendships? Committed to the political change which never came. Which, indeed, was not to come for another 40 years?

It is gone, the world we shared.

We last met 10 years ago, on our last visit to South Africa. Now you both live in a frail care centre; ironically part of a fortified complex. Val and Edward drive us across from Pretoria. It is late autumn with periods of sharp, clear sunlight punctuated by the last sheeting rains of summer. The highways with all their cars and reckless drivers are obscured by the spray, making it hard to see where we are going. The soil and dirt roads turn to red mud, the unmistakable red of the African high veld. That at least has not changed.

So we meet again. Your Parkinson's is now

advanced and you cannot sit up at all. You move your head and arms with difficulty. Michael says you are confused and not able to communicate much today. But he thinks you know we are coming.

I kneel down next to your bed, taking your hand. And you know me immediately, using the pet name which only people from that time call me. "Margie," you say, in that stubbornly upper class English accent, your blue eyes lighting up, "and dear John. How wonderful to see you!" Michael has put photographs on the walls round your bed hoping to help you hold on to the memories slipping out of your grasp. He is trying to throw you the life belt, which was not there at Mazeppa Bay. He loves you so much.

We talk as two women who have lived in the same vanished world. We share almost nothing in the present. We can only meet in the past. In the world which no longer exists. There is an instant feeling of connection between us. The conversation becomes general and starts to pass you by. "Michael is a darling man," you say quietly, "but he does have a terribly loud voice! Speak up Margie dear, I can't catch what you're saying." I am filled with affection for you. Gratitude for the loving support you gave us in that long ago tragedy. And for today. Your humour is still there. You are manifestly still you. Because our shared world exists only inside our own heads, the loss of your short term memory does not matter. It is, in fact, an advantage. Your mind is not full of all the myriad things which clutter mine. The years between then and now have vanished. All that matters is now.

Back in Pretoria Val says: "You are much better at talking to someone like her than I am." I just don't know what to say. I reply without thinking: "It is my job." But that meeting was not about my job. It was not about knowing how to talk to someone with memory loss. It was an intensely real connection between old friends who shared a vanished world. It was wonderful. It was a gift to treasure.

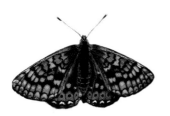

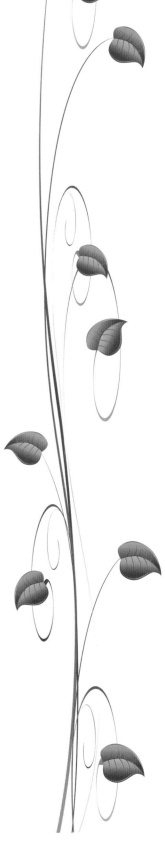

Time!

Bill Wilson

Bill Wilson was born in Coventry in 1950 and attended King Henry VIII school. On leaving, he joined the Royal Marines. His love of all sports has never left him and he was part of the 'team' that took his daughter to international level as a sprinter. Bill is married to Pat and is now an ambassador for the Alzheimer's Society. He lives for every day, challenging Alzheimer's to put another hurdle in his way that he surely will surmount.

Thank goodness for dementia and its 'hosts' – we who live it 24/7. Strange, you must be thinking, but personally, I have accepted my 'beast'. That description is another story, you must ask me about it another time!

Time to me is a friend. My life, by choice, now revolves about dementia. I write constantly about my life. I travel to talk on how I tour the country alongside my 'fellow hosts'. Time now is my employer. I find that I will, first thing in the morning, plan my day to what I want and not be dictated by the 'system', as I am like most people with the beast. I have a family so a lot of my former 'jobs' are no longer safe, shall I say, in my hands – monetary transactions for example, over the phone. So what can I do?

I can do things that I did 20, 30 years ago - mix cement and build a small wall. I did things like that before I was 'inducted' into this very elite family and that has, in all honesty, given, in a funny kind of a way, me my life again that I lived and enjoyed so many years ago. My memories. And as everyone who has dementia lives and hopefully loves, recalling our former years, so now we all have time on our hands. I for one – I am thankful.

Using the past

Faith Gibson

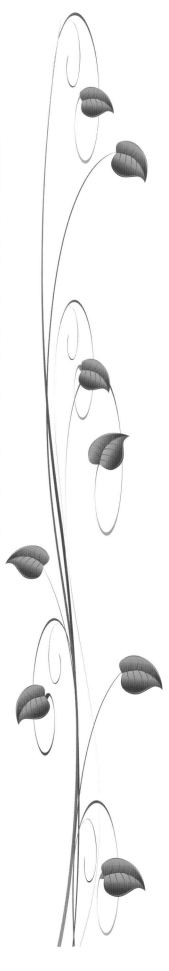

"The future is not ours
We hold the present by a brittle thread
It is the past that is in our hearts" (anon)

Most of us experience time as transitory, ephemeral and on occasion even threatening. Time for all of us of whatever age is frequently perplexing. How we perceive it seems to vary across the age span and whether our present living circumstances and state of health are satisfactory or not. Very young children find its passing slow and endless; middle aged people find it hectic, even frenetic; younger older people perceive it as accelerating; and many very old and frail people finding time interminable will say they have lived long enough and "it's time to be away". No matter how we define time, try to contain it, enjoy or endure it, as time is customarily parcelled out in minutes, days, weeks and years we are its slaves rather than its masters. While we may go to extraordinary lengths to persuade ourselves and others that we are the captains of our souls and the masters of our fate, we know that it was never thus nor ever can be.

Consequently we are all in the same boat. Whether or not we happen to be experiencing any of the conditions loosely labelled dementia, time is beyond everyone's control and how we perceive it will be determined by diverse factors only one of which will be our cognitive competence. The tendency to forget recently acquired knowledge and experience more readily, and recall earlier memories more easily, is a common characteristic of most dementias. The impaired ability to recall recent times, places, people, information and events causes enormous problems for adequately maintaining autonomy, control, independence, security and well-being. But the relatively uncompromised ability to retain long-term memory, at least for a time despite dementia, can prove a resource in the present. If long-stored memories, 'the past that is in our hearts', can be revived or reactivated, such memories can provide a bridge to the here and now of time present.

We do well to remember that we all hold the present by nothing more than a brittle thread – a thread which at any moment and in myriad ways may be easily broken. While for all of us, regardless of our level of cognitive functioning, the future is not ours and is more or less impossible to know, to predict or to control in other than crude and unpredictable ways.

For the past 25 years or more I have devoted much time to persuading people that the past, accessed through memory and imagination, is an incomparable resource for most, though not all, people as they age. Furthermore, while memory is a rich goldmine that is potentially available to every one at any age, just awaiting exploration, particularly by means of reminiscence and linked creative activities, it can be of enormous value for people who develop dementia. I still believe this to be true and indicative empirical research as well as much clinical experience supports this conviction (Woods *et al* 2005, Bohlmeijer *et al* 2007).

I wish that more health and social care professionals as well as hard pressed family carers, volunteers and friends would utilise this cheap, accessible, low risk, mostly enjoyable and widely acceptable resource – and not just for people with dementia. Mining the past brings instantaneous pleasure and satisfaction to those who engage in reminiscence, life review, life story work, guided or independent autobiographical writing or other forms of narrative exploration. Such memory excavation may be a private or shared activity, undertaken alone, with a companion or in small sociable groups. Much has been written about the objectives, techniques and outcomes of these various biographical approaches.

These details do not need to be rehearsed here, although I do urge readers to explore the contribution which such approaches can make to present well-being and mutual satisfaction. The desirable outcomes include developing and sustaining relationships, giving pleasure, decreasing boredom and enriching communication between people (Birren and Cochran 2001, Gibson 2004, Gibson 2006, Haight 2007, Schweitzer and Bruce 2008). I am assuming readers will either already be familiar with such literature or will explore it for themselves. Some guidance is given in the references listed below.

Recalling memories of the past enriches the present. Reminiscence is essentially a personal, although often sociable, experience which takes place in the here and now. Whether it is limited to private rumination, is shared in conversation with other people or is given substance in writing, drawing, painting or other artistic forms, all these activities take place in the present. Once memories are put outside oneself in such ways they become more accessible and can be revisited, remembered and reconstructed. They become available for further exploration and a source of future satisfaction.

Birren J, Cochran K (2001) *Telling the Stories of Life through Guided Autobiography Groups*. Health Professions Press, Baltimore.

Bohlmeijer E, Roemer M, Cuijpers P, Smit F (2007) The effects of reminiscence on psychological well-being in older adults: a meta-analysis. *Aging and Mental Health* 11(3) 291-300.

Gibson F (2004) *The Past in the present: Reminiscence in health and social care*. Health Professions Press, Baltimore.

Gibson F (2006) *Reminiscence and Recall: A practical guide to reminiscence work*. Age Concern, London.

Haight B, Haight B (2007) *The Handbook of Structured Life Review*. Health Professions Press, Baltimore.

Schweitzer P, Bruce E (2008) *Remembering Yesterday, Caring Today*. Jessica Kingsley Publishers, London.

Woods B, Spector A, Jones C, Orrell M, Davies S (2005), Reminiscence therapy for dementia, *Cochrane Database of Systematic Reviews* Issue 1, Art. No. CD001120.

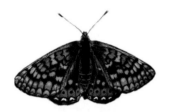

08:04

Are the happy times to be allowed once more?

Päivi Topo

Päivi Topo, PhD is an adjunct professor in sociology of medicine in the University of Helsinki and is currently working as an academy research fellow for the Academy of Finland. She has been involved in research on people with memory problems for over 10 years and has published on ethical issues in dementia care and in research involving people with dementia, care quality, use of technology in supporting people with dementia and their carers, and the importance of psychosocial and physical environments for the well-being of people with memory problems. She has co-edited a book with professor Britt Östlund entitled *Dementia, Design and Technology*, published by IOS press in 2009.

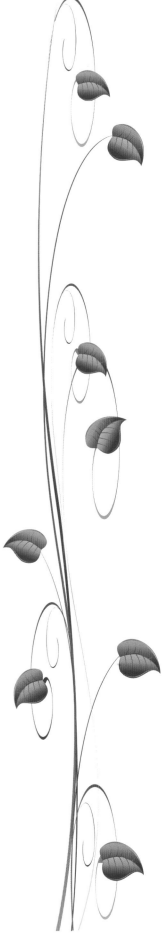

Some years ago we carried out a study based on observations of people with dementia who were either living in residential care or were using a dementia day care centre. During the observations it became obvious that one of the real challenges for the care workers and family members is how to accept the subjective reality of persons with memory problems. I'm not sure if this is mainly a matter of lack of knowledge of the impact of dementia on a human being or whether it is somehow associated with difficulties we all have in facing vulnerability in others and in ourselves. Our western idea of time as a linear concept can make this even harder because illnesses causing dementia diminish one's ability to work with such a linear concept of time.

Below is a rough translation of our Finnish study (Topo *et al* 2007). It is an episode that took place in a nursing home where a woman, here referred to as Mrs Heinonen, had been living for a couple of years.

Mrs Heinonen has finished her supper and asks a carer, "Is this paid for?"

The carer: "Yes, it has been paid."

Mrs Heinonen: "Has my husband left already?"

The carer: "Do you remember that your husband has died. You have been a widow for a long time." Mrs Heinonen is astonished: "Now - I'm very confused."

The carer tries to suggest to Mrs Heinonen the contemporary time by pointing to flowers in a vase on a window bench and photographs of the residents next to the flowers. Mrs Heinonen is quiet but after a while she looks at the carer and says, "Thank you. It is good that I asked you."

The carer leaves. Mrs Heinonen stays still and seems to be very thoughtful. After some 20 minutes she heaves a deep sigh and says to herself, "It is so hard."

This episode raised many questions in my mind. Why remind the person every day about the great losses they have experienced? What is the right time and what is the wrong time? Is subjective time less relevant than objective time? Could it help all of us if we could sometimes give up the idea of linear time which has actually been developed to serve the interests of the industrial society? Why not let people with memory problems live their happy times again?

Topo P, Sormunen S, Saarikalle K, Räikkönen O, Eloniemi-Sulkava U. Daily encounters in dementia care. An observational study of care quality from the client's perspective. *STAKES*, research reports 162, Helsinki 2007. (Abstract in English)

08:05

Under the Comet
15 May 1997

Peter C Jackson

Peter Jackson has been a journalist, editor and consultant in organisational communication who, in retirement, continues to write and edit prose, poetry and drama. In 1997 (the year of the Hale-Bopp comet) his mother Edie was admitted to a psychiatric ward in the first stages of Alzheimer's disease. He says: "This poem reflects some of my daily visits to that bleak, soulless place where helpers with limited training tried to cope with a milling crowd of people in various stages of dementia. Fortunately, the last years of Edie's long life were spent in the tranquil surroundings of a superb specialist home run by the Augustinian Order of nuns, but it is the vision of that grey, unforgiving ward (now demolished) that returns from the past to haunt my imagination." This poem won second prize in the Alzheimer's Society Poetry Competition, judged by Roger McGough, in 2009.

Florence, Rose and Alice strut
the ward's grey catwalk
in relentless pursuit of freedom.
In the crook of Florence's arm
Is a bear with a bagged head
– proof against toy thieves.

Rose chassés between her sticks
as the gramophone spins
her latest cha cha pupil
up the linoleum street
to where the locked door
(PLEASE RING FOR
ADMITTANCE)
keeps the world at bay.

Alice fingers her dressing gown
(ALL GARMENTS MUST BE
CLEARLY MARKED)
and eyes the bowling green
through the Sluice Room window.
Another rink will soon be ending
and, with more teas to prepare,
she hurries to the kitchen.

Was it today that lunch came round
two minutes since or
when they lived at home and
mother called them in from play?
Listen – she's calling now, and
they must turn and tread
the grey linoleum once more.

Upon the dayroom wall
the season's written out with
weather, date and menus
brightly spread.
Just like those pictures
on the classroom wall.
Is that today or
sixty years ago?

The words are Wash and
Toilet and Injection.
But what of Faith and
Hope and Love?
How can they find
the meaning of rejection
when cells that gave that
meaning life are gone?

Light years above the Sluice Room door
Hale-Bopp shines on;
Predictable, remote.
Behind its forked tail
Florence, Rose and Alice
strut the Milky Way,
curlers and stardust in their hair,
into a brighter dawn,
a farther shore,
where bears range free
and dancers spin
and every wood that's bowled
touches the jack.

08:06

Time is a great healer
when sleeping dogs are left to lie

Ian James

Ian James (PhD), is a consultant in clinical psychology, and Head of Newcastle Challenging Behaviour Service, Northumberland Tyne and Wear NHS Trust. He has published widely on the use of psychotherapy with people with dementia and staff training. He is the Associate Editor of *Behavioural and Cognitive Psychotherapy*, the UK CBT journal.

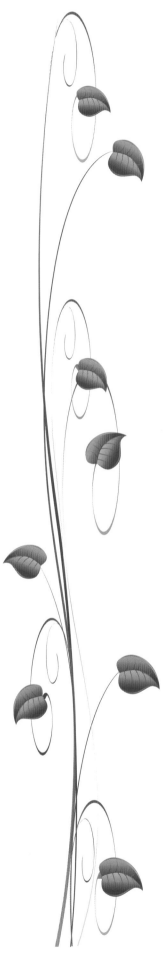

Hard Times

(i)

Each year, in early December
Grandma would oblige by falling over
and dislocating something

In hospital, on Christmas Day
all the family would visit
Sit around the bed and gobble up her dinner

(iii)

If we could have afforded a bath
We would have had the best. A fine one
Iron. Broad as a bed, deep as the ocean
Standing on winged feet, proud as a lion

And oh, what coal we would have stored in it.
Nuggets, big as babies' heads, still blinking
   in the daylight
Black as wedding-boots, so polished you
   could see your face in them

And oh, what stories we might have told.
Seated round the hearth on winter nights
The fire crackling, the flames leaping.
Amber liquor sparkling in crystal glasses.

Unfortunately, we were too poor to
   know stories.

– From *Hard Times* by Roger McGough
(sections 1 and 3)

Roger McGough's poem reminds me that our past is complex territory, and humour can be a cloak hiding distress, hardship and pain. This is an important point for me to remember as a clinician, for often I am required to ask highly personal questions about people's histories (Did you get on with your mother? Can you tell me about the death of your twin sister?). As such, I have become more cautious when undertaking 'life story' work, because of the traumatic experiences one sometimes uncovers (eg parental abuse, giving up a child for adoption, a difficult divorce).

In my experience, in most situations when a difficult event is discussed, initially people tend to say they've either resolved or forgotten the issue. However, every so often I am aware that the reviewing process unintentionally reawakens problems. For example, in some circumstances one can cause people to engage in a negative reappraisal of an episode. Consider the case of Mary, who had divorced in her 30s due to suffering physical abuse from her husband. As a younger woman, she was confident and determined, and was prepared to stand up for herself and protect her child from her violent husband. However, years later, and with the onset of her dementia, she found this part of her life difficult to come to terms with. When reminded of the divorce via the questions I asked her, she could no longer

111

remember the details of the abuse. Hence, all she recalled was the fact she'd left a man she had made a vow to stay with "... at the altar!". Her realisation of the latter, and hazy memory for the context of the separation, was now causing her great distress.

Having outlined my reservations about taking histories, I have to say that I believe 'life-story' work plays an important role in helping us to understand people's needs. Nevertheless, I think that we need to highlight the pros and cons of such approaches, and pay more attention to 'resolution' approaches that seek to deal with the re-emergence of problematic memories (Haight & Burnside 1993).

Haight BK, Burnside I (1993) Reminiscence and life review: explaining the difference. *Archives of Psychiatric Nursing 7* 91-98.
McGough R (1992) Hard times. *Defying Gravity*. Viking, London.

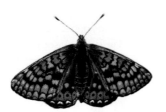

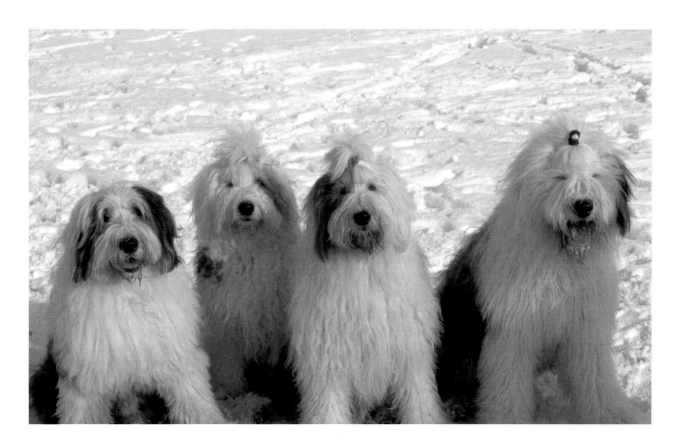

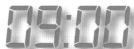

Pastimes

09:01

Busy doing nothing

Claire Craig

Claire Craig is a senior lecturer and researcher in occupational therapy at Sheffield Hallam University. Much of her work has focused on the arts and the opportunities that they offer people with dementia. She lives in Yorkshire with her husband Neil and Eddie the dog and spends most of her spare time walking in Derbyshire.

As an occupational therapist time and time usage fascinate me. The decisions we make about how we use the hours of the day define who we are, reflect our priorities and have a significant bearing on our health and well-being. When we manage to get the balance right our lives sit in equilibrium. We feel sufficiently challenged to be stimulated but not exhausted. The opposite is also true. Too many things to do and too little time to do these in result in stress and exhaustion; too much time and too few things to do result in boredom.

I see both extremes in the context of my work with people with dementia. Large care home settings with few resources and task-based cultures. On the one hand staff speak of being overwhelmed by the number of activities they need to perform and of being under constant pressure. The idea of spending time having a drink with a resident and sitting and talking is uncomfortable. "Time is for work and not for socialising," one person told me; "The only way to cope or to avoid burn out is to emotionally tune out," another staff member said.

On the other hand I see residents, people with dementia, sitting for hour after hour with little or no stimulation and with nothing to do. How they use time is dictated by the institution. This is yet another area of their lives that is beyond their control. Denied the opportunity to carry out the everyday tasks that members of staff are so concerned they don't have time to perform, they have to wait for pockets of 'organised activities' as and when they are able to happen. Rather than meaningful activities being spontaneous they are 'timetabled' into specific slots. Even the timing of these can undo any therapeutic potential. For instance hand and nail care just before lunch when in fact it would be more appropriate to offer this following a bath.

Yet it does not have to be this way. I have also visited settings where people with dementia and staff work together in partnership and those everyday tasks are transformed into opportunities for meaningful engagement. Faded timetables of 'activity sessions' to slot people into are a thing of the past. Spontaneity is the order of the day and meaningful use of time pervades the culture. The results speak for themselves. Time is something to be shared. Staff are no longer overwhelmed and residents are no longer 'busy doing nothing'.

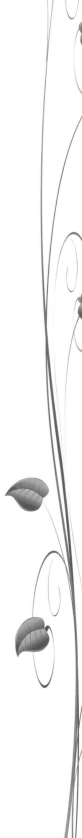

Timing dementia

Wendy Hulko

Dr Wendy Hulko is Assistant Professor of Social Work at Thompson Rivers University in Kamloops, British Columbia, Canada and a qualified health researcher with the Centre for Research on Personhood in Dementia at the University of British Columbia in Vancouver, BC. A former residential care aide, hospital social worker and policy advisor for Ontario's Alzheimer Strategy, Wendy currently applies her passion for social justice and commitment to ageing and dementia care to research and teaching. She is currently conducting grounded theory research on indigenous world views on memory loss and memory care in later life in conjunction with two decision-makers from the Interior Health Authority and elders from two local First Nation bands.

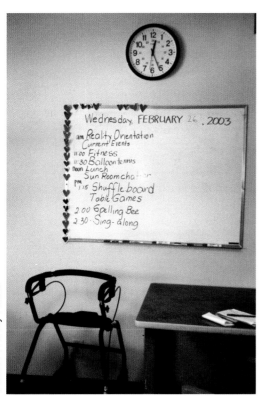

Photo: Wendy Hulko

This photo was taken at a dementia day programme in Toronto, Canada in February 2003 during grounded theory research into subjective experiences of dementia and the intersections of race, class, ethnicity and gender (see Hulko, in press). The schedule of activities, starting with reality orientation at 10am and ending with a sing-a-long at 2.30pm, is a visual testament to the way in which the provision of care is so often centred on keeping bodies in motion and making sure that people are occupied at all times (see Katz 2000). The walking frame indicates a body in need of assistance to get to the activities on the schedule and the note pad and paper remind us of the importance of recording events, such as the performance of activities of daily living (ADLs) and instrumental activities of daily living (IADLs). Although there is no human subject in the photo, the image of ageing that is depicted is one of physical and cognitive impairment and the prescription appears to be programmed activity. It is telling that, according to the schedule, there is no time to discuss shared experiences of dementia during this dementia day programme; and this was certainly not the focus of the 'sun room chatter' after lunch that day. Talking with the people for whom one cares may be viewed as too challenging or uncomfortable by workers and as too idle or futile by their managers, unless the worker assists with ADLs at the same time.

Hulko W (in press). From 'not a big deal' to 'hellish': Experiences of older people with dementia. *Journal of Aging Studies* 23(3). doi:10.1016/j.jaging.2007.11.002.
Katz S (2000). Busy bodies: Activity, aging, and the management of everyday life. *Journal of Aging Studies* 14(2), 135-152.

Your time

Sue Benson

Sue Benson has been editor of the *Journal of Dementia Care* since its launch in 1993, and is passionate about the potential of the arts to improve communication with and well-being of people with dementia. Following a degree in English at Hull University she trained and worked as a state registered nurse in London, then as an editor on health service journals including Nursing Mirror. She is also a musician, singer and Morris dancer.

I'm trying to give you back your time
That's the plan
First, slow down
Take time out to become calm
Slow my pace.

Approach gently
Choose words with care
Slowly, clearly, warmly
"I've come to invite you…"

Your time as a dancer
As you watch, your body remembers
Responds
Neurons make the same connections
As if you were dancing too
It's not such a passive activity.

Your time in the theatre
Makes you critical of 'entertainment'
But when skilled actors make contact
Pride returns.

Your time in church
Hymn words remembered, sung clearly
Hot iron on starched white linen.

Your time as a parent, grandparent
Mrs Tiggywinkle
When We Were Very Young.

These can bring the reward I crave
Smiles, spoken words
I plan, prepare, manage
Hardest, most vital is to slow down
Find inner calm.

Still working on it.

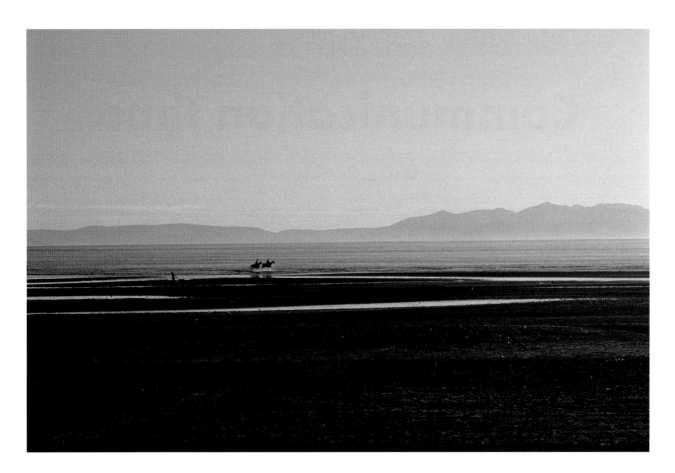

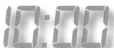

Making good use of time

Communication time

Barry Pankhurst

Barry Pankhurst is 62 and was diagnosed with mixed dementia/Alzheimer's in 2005. He lives in Indonesia with his Indonesian wife and extended family. He has lived there for the past 16 years and has not lived in the UK for over 26 years as his past job (master baker and confectioner advisor) kept him continuously travelling around the Middle and Far East, training clients in all aspects of the baking industry. He returned to live in Indonesia as his wife could not get accustomed to the English way of life.

Given my own somewhat different situation of having mixed dementia/Alzheimer's and living in a small village community in Indonesia, where I have no local Alzheimer's society or day centre support and no one to talk to in my own native English, communication time using the internet, emails, and instant messaging has become of major importance to me in fighting my illness. I must do all of this completely alone as I have no one to help me with typing or any computer work.

Prior to being diagnosed with my illness, some three and a half years ago, I had many Indonesian English language teacher friends who would come to my home regularly to spend time practising their English conversation. I would also visit their schools and give talks to the students about the differences of customs, cultures, traditions, and communication skills using English. But then I started to realise I was having a big problem when trying to translate words and phrases from Indonesian into good English. Trying to remember and find the right words to use was becoming increasingly difficult, so I had to stop giving my school lectures. When I explained why to the teachers and about my Alzheimer's and dementia, they all disappeared in a cloud of dust never to be seen again, which is basically due to the fact that apart from my doctor/specialist, nobody where I live has ever heard of or understands anything about dementia or Alzheimer's. It was even a problem for my wife and her family to try and understand as the perception of people here is that a curse has been put on me by black magic – voodoo – or that it's an infectious disease.

Having lost all my so-called friends, I started to concentrate all my time and efforts using my computer, communicating with my family in England. Then I contacted the UK Alzheimer's Society and Alzheimer's

Forum, which opened up a whole new world for me as I could communicate with people who had understanding of my illness and correspond with fellow sufferers, one of whom has become a very close, albeit distant, friend. We regularly send each other emails, photographs, and send recorded talks to each other via email. We have also spent a lot of time making video and two-way conversation recordings about how we cope with our illness and the problems arising from dementia. I then put the recordings all together as one continuous recording, which is then put on the Alzheimer's Forum website for other sufferers to watch and listen to. It's a case of sufferers taking the time communicating together and hopefully helping their fellows.

But my communication time doesn't stop there as I communicate with Alzheimer's Forum almost every day, sending articles and poems that are put on the website. Occasionally, if Ellie who runs the website is online, we sit and have a chat using the instant messenger, which really is quality time in communication for me that I now desperately need. Even with all this going on, I have still been keeping a daily diary of how my illness is slowly progressing and typed it all down into an autobiography of my dementia, with all the past memories that now rush into my brain of my youth, family and past job as a globe-trotting master baker and confectioner. I continuously look for ways to use my time and keep my brain active, and have just finished writing my own book of Kriss Kross puzzles, conundrums, memory exercises, and poems specifically for people with early to mid stage dementia and their families.

So, yes, spending my time communicating to others has become very important to me as a way of fighting dementia. We must be prepared to push ourselves to our limits to keep our brains working.

In the nick of time

Graham Browne

Graham Browne was diagnosed with Pick's disease in 2006 at the age of 49. Determined to fight it and not just sit and waste away, he joined the Towner club in Brighton. He is now an Alzheimer's ambassador for the national office of the Alzheimer's Society and works as a volunteer for the Brighton and Hove branch.

They say time is a great healer, but whoever said that could never have had dementia. On that fateful day in June 2006, when I was diagnosed with Pick's disease, I realised that I would have plenty of time on my hands. I was no longer the breadwinner. What would I do?

We had gone to see the consultant expecting bad news, but all the better if it was good. But we had never expected the scale of what we were told.

We went home, both stunned and numb. My wife, Debs, found a club, the Towner Club for younger people with dementia, on the local Brighton and Hove Alzheimer's website.

Within a week of a home visit, I was accepted and since then I have not looked back. I now spend the time I would have spent sitting at home attending meetings, doing talks at universities and helping second year GP students. I am doing a trainer's course.

My diary is busy every week now, and I have no time to waste. I hope what I'm doing will help future people with dementia. Debs and I work hard together – and laugh every day to get through it. So my advice to anyone is – don't sit and mope. Get out and help yourself and others.

I do not have a clock to sit and watch time go by. But the best time is when we spend our time with our very special grandson, Kyle. We also make time to be together.

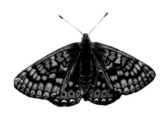

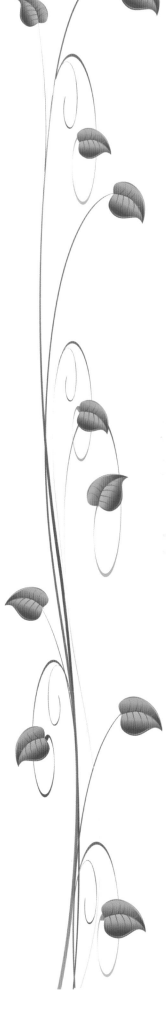

10:03

Reflections on experiences of time in a longitudinal study

Errollyn Bruce

Errollyn Bruce is a lecturer with the Bradford Dementia Group at the University of Bradford. She is interested in experiences of dementia and ways to promote well-being among people with dementia and those who care for them.

Time plays a big part in experiences of dementia. This is true for researchers, practitioners and carers who look at dementia from the outside as well as those inside dementia. From outside we can see that people's performance varies from time to time, and that they change as their condition progresses. Conversations with people inside dementia suggest that they too have considerable awareness of these fluctuations and changes. A longitudinal study of well-being in people with moderate to severe dementia provided an opportunity for conversations with the general theme 'How are you doing?' (Bruce *et al* 2002) and many people mentioned changes over time (Clare *et al* 2008 a & b). For example, one person said, "My brain goes to sleep sometimes," echoing Margaret Eleanor, interviewed by a colleague in Canada, who said: "I go in and out" (Purves *et al* 2000). Bill Nichols was aware of major changes in himself: "I used to be a bloke that knew different things and all that... I've lost it... really lost it."

At times what people said showed that they felt that it was not them, but the world that had changed. In a sense they are right – as Tom Kitwood argued so forcefully, the world does change when you have dementia (Kitwood 1997). Muriel Broadbent, who spent much of her time walking arm in arm with a man who was not her husband, commented: "It wouldn't be too bad if it wasn't so strange." Muriel's dementia meant moving to live with strangers in an unfamiliar place and being treated differently by other people. When Molly Sharp said, "Those times have gone – people don't act the same, do they, these days," was she just referring to social changes over a lifetime, or did her comment also spring from her more recent experience of changes associated with dementia?

The longitudinal study meant repeated visits – up to eight over two years – which allowed us to get to know people and learn how to communicate with each individual. We were also able to hear what they had to say at different times and in different moods, and observe how the conversations changed for people experiencing a rapid decline. We learned to spot good moments for conversation, though it was not always possible to get the timing right, as a field note illustrates: "I taped a sticky conversation with Bill where he said very little... later he approached me, and talked at some length about a time when he had 'nearly topped himself'... but I couldn't tape this without interrupting the intensity of the moment." Nonetheless, the advantages of a longitudinal study were reflected in the material – many of the later conversations were richer than first ones.

Of the many time-related issues that arose during the study, two stand out – an altered sense of time, and outpacing. Alterations in awareness of time often contributed to behaviour that upset and baffled others. Mabel Hamilton's family visited very frequently and sometimes she said "My family come to see me...they're very good" but more often she felt lonely and abandoned and would say, "Why don't they come to see me?" When we took account of her variable sense of time, what she said made sense. The vividness of distant memories, and their coherence and consistency, brings the distant past closer, whereas recent events are often foggy and faded by comparison. Sometimes the past conflicts confusingly with barely remembered details of the present. Jill Brennan was puzzled about the whereabouts of the family that she recalled so clearly: "I wish I knew what's happened to my family. I ha' have a queer feeling of thinking… that they can't all be living anyway… Because I was the youngest… it had probably happened longer ago than I am thinking of… so I doubt whether any of them are living."

But her doubts ebbed and flowed. On recalling her sister's musical abilities she said: "Something I've heard recently, and I thought 'Well I think she's knocking around'." Some people resolve a tangled sense of time by blending past and present. Alice Baker often said, "I'm waiting for me mum, she'll be here soon," and was one of many who seemed to take comfort from revisiting the times when her mother was never far away.

On many occasions during the study I was reminded that the world of those outside dementia tends to go too fast for those inside. The risk of this 'outpacing' was ever-present. People with dementia need extra time to gather their thoughts and express themselves in words. Bill Nichols commented: "Well I have slowed down now… it's too much, you know." But we too need extra time to get to know people as individuals and understand how best to foster connections with them. Few people in our study could remember who we were, but most could pick up on subtle cues. Having time to get to know them made it easier for us to provide the cues that

signal familiarity and being known. If people with dementia are to participate fully and tell us what they need us to know, professional practice must be prepared to slacken its pace.

Longitudinal studies are valued for being able to follow individuals through time, and explore changes. They are particularly suited to phenomena that are inherently extended across time. Dementia is, but unpredictably so, and tends to be longer-running than longitudinal studies. The two-year time period was a luxury, yet too short to give us an extensive understanding of how and why things changed for each person as dementia ran its course. We really needed to know more about both what had happened before, and what was going to happen next, to judge how a person was faring at any given point in time. Time is expensive. Finding funding for long-running qualitative work that follows people with dementia over time requires researchers who are committed, persistent, and above all, generous with their time.

Bruce F, Surr C, Tibbs MA (2002) *A special kind of care: Improving well-being in people living with dementia*. MHA Care Group, Derby. Available from www.bradford.ac.uk/acad/health/dementia
Clare L, Rowlands J, Bruce E, Surr C, Downs M (2008a) The experience of living with dementia in residential care: an interpretive phenomenological analysis. *The Gerontologist* 48 (6) 711-20.
Clare L, Rowlands J, Bruce E, Surr C, Downs M (2008b) 'I don't do like I used to do': a grounded theory approach to conceptualising awareness in people with moderate to severe dementia living in long-term care. *Social Science & Medicine* 66 (11) 2366-2377.
Kitwood T (1997) Dementia Reconsidered. Open University Press, Buckingham.
Purves B, O'Connor D, Perry J A (2000) *From patient to person: Changing the lens in dementia care.* ITServices/Telestudios, University of British Columbia, Vancouver (CD-rom presentation).

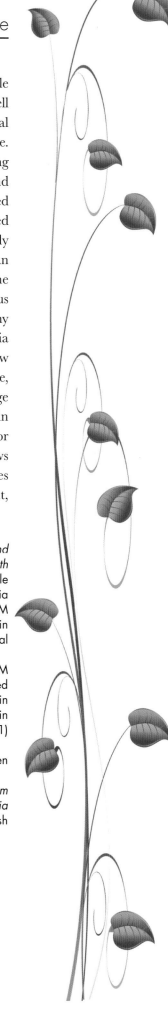

10:04

Time to say goodbye

Linda Hunt

Linda Hunt was in social work practice for several years and then spent 10 years in an academic appointment before becoming a senior advisor and then assistant chief inspector of social work in Scotland. She recently completed her period as chair of the Board of Circle, Scotland. Her published work has focused primarily on work with people who have alcohol problems, group and organisational issues and the impact of earlier trauma in late life.

"I had already said goodbye."

I was surprised by this part of our conversation when I was talking with a friend a few weeks after the death of her husband. It set me thinking about one aspect of time, for those concerned for a loved one who is becoming progressively impaired by dementia. My friend's experience illustrates the point.

She had lived with, and cared for, her husband for 10 years following his diagnosis. His physical fitness and highly developed social skills enabled him to stay active and to some extent involved in family and friendship networks for some of those years. He remained his gentle and thoughtful self although his uncertainty and confusion became increasingly apparent. Her life changed more and more as home, relationships and social activities had to be adjusted to take account of his increasing handicap. Many of the things they had shared together had to be given up as she said 'goodbye' to aspects of their relationship and their life together.

Eventually when his restlessness and anxiety became intense and his ability to know where he was and who he was reduced further, he was admitted to residential care. My friend spent time with him daily for many months. She took him swimming, which he loved, and brought him home at weekends. She soon had to face the fact that he did not recognise "home" and was upset at being there. It was so difficult for them both to manage these visits that they were discontinued. She went on visiting him as, over a period of 18 months or so, he came to need more and more personal care and was less and less able to communicate with her or to recognise her as his wife.

Saying the last goodbye to someone we have cared about is always a sad and painful experience. We need to take our time over coming to terms with our feelings (which may be quite mixed) and our sense of loss. In these circumstances we say to each other "time is a great healer", and in a general way that is true. But my friend, like many others with a family member with dementia, was saying her last goodbye to her husband stage by stage over a period of more than 12 years as, little by little, his ability to be her husband and father of their children in the ways that had earlier characterised him diminished and disappeared. Time does not seem like a healer in this situation, where 'goodbye' is experienced stage by painful stage and we do not know how many more painful stages there will be. The present time is emotionally difficult and the future looks as if it holds further difficulties.

We talk of 'time to say goodbye' as a way of indicating that the moment has come for something to end, but in my friend's situation (and that of many other carers) the 'time' is not one, but a continually recurring moment. The raw feeling that comes with 'goodbye' is a repeated experience, as element after element of the relationship is lost for the present time and for the future. The feeling can become the more painful if there is some awareness that there are going to be yet more goodbyes as the horizons and the capacity of the spouse, parent or sibling become more limited. At the same time, because the person is physically present and a central part of their lives, family members may feel miserably guilty about engaging emotionally in the process of saying goodbye (of letting go). However, although it does not bring closure, perhaps it can help begin the healing process, That is what happened to my friend.

"Take your time" is what we say when we are trying to encourage someone who is experiencing difficulty in speaking about or coming to terms with powerful emotion. We usually mean 'don't hurry' but we can also be encouraging the person to *give time* to sorting out the difficulty. In the case of people living with the increasing dementia of a family member, encouragement to give time to the many stages of 'goodbye' could be helpful.

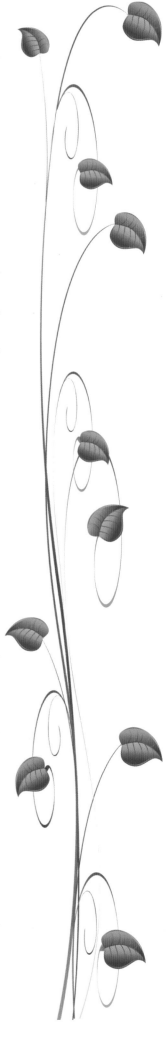

10:05

Using time fully

Andy Barker

Dr Andy Barker works in Hampshire, where he has been a consultant in old age psychiatry for the past 10 years.

A patient of mine once said that up until retirement it was as though you had to live two lives, but after, you could get on with just your own. This rang bells for me, juggling my personal and professional lives, struggling with my life/work balance. I let my personal life get pressured by work and other commitments but want, some day, to be able to have more time to reflect on the more important things in life.

If dementia can be appropriately described as a living bereavement for carers, it must be like living through death for the person. The dissolution of awareness and 'self' that dementia often brings holds a morbid curiosity for me.

As long as I can remember, I have been fascinated by consciousness and life's purpose. As a child brought up in a Christian household this meant wondering who or what it was I was praying to, and what the meaning of life was. As my religious leanings have changed, towards Buddhist philosophy, I have become more preoccupied with what it means to live a good life, and the nature of reality and consciousness.

In my professional life I meet people with dementia in their latter years, who have plenty of time in their day for reflection but for whom there is an urgency in finding meaning and for whom the cognitive capacity for reflection is diminishing.

People often ask me whether it is depressing doing the work I do. Well, yes, and no.

Yes, partly because of being confronted by the tragedy of losses for the individuals concerned, but also because I see so many wasted lives. So many people who have postponed their aspirations and ambitions until retirement, but find their plans disintegrate. The future I fear.

No, because I am reminded every day of how fortunate I am, in the many little things I would otherwise take for granted. I am also privileged to do a job that lets me into the heart of people's lives, joys and tragedies, and to learn from them.

I have met many remarkable people struggling with the implications of progressive dementia, and I hope I have learnt much from them. Some who have built their self-identity on the basis of impermanent foundations which they cling to with increasing desperation. Some who have found a peace and a simplicity in life which I envy.

For the moment, I juggle my desire for reflection and to live fully in the moment, with my responsibilities in planning for a secure future as husband and father. My work with people with dementia allows me the opportunity to learn from others who are living for better and worse through a decline in consciousness, and reminds me to reflect on the importance of using time fully now. And I hope for us all to have a meaningful life; in Buddhist terms, to continue searching for truth and practising compassion.

10:06

Time stood still!

James McKillop

James McKillop is married with four children. He led an ordinary sort of life and his life was his family. The family had a rough time before diagnosis as his behaviour had changed. Luckily with treatment and support they are now back to a family unit. With the support he gets from his family, his medication and dedicated support workers, he now plays an active part in the community and is on many committees, some unconnected with dementia eg learning difficulties. He gives many talks to encourage others with the illness, and carers, to make the best of their lives.

I read that when you are about to die, your life flashes past before your eyes. I wasn't at death's door (though I felt like it later) but this is what happened within a few seconds.

I was suddenly much younger, back into my mid twenties. I used to go to what was called a 'mental hospital' in those days with my mother. We went to visit her sister's sister-in-law. It was awful, the place smelled with odours of cooking, body odour, urine and faecal waste. There were wails and shrieks and people shambling and shuffling about. Old ladies, drooling at the mouth would grab my arm and claim me for their son. Others asked me to take them home. Some rocked themselves in corners and muttered unintelligible mantras. It was bedlam. I felt like Dante on the earlier part of his journey. All all I knew was that the patients had dementia.

My life then fast forwarded 10 years. I was now working as a hospital auditor and spent a lot of time in long-stay hospitals where dementia was prevalent. The hospitals catered for up to three thousand patients. Nothing had really changed, but this time I saw more of the staff and noticed their dedication and the (unpleasant) conditions they worked under.

I was jolted back to the present, the consultant's words ringing and echoing in my ear: "I am sorry but you have dementia."

I was devastated. All I could see was a big black hole and my life had come to a crushing end. When would I be admitted to hospital? Would I get visitors who would squirm at the surroundings and my appearance? Would I have to ring a bell to let people know I was coming? I was terrified. I drove home, my mind in turmoil. I should not have been allowed to drive after the diagnosis; I was in no fit state. I spent many months at home, cut off from society and deeply depressed. I had reached the stage of being ready for a care home.

So I am now in the present.

My life nine years later is very enjoyable, yes I repeat enjoyable. So what happened. It is a long story and I will not steal my own thunder by saying it here, in case the reader happens to hear me and my presentation. Brenda, a worker from Alzheimer Scotland, came to visit and briefly she coaxed me back into society. She persuaded me to talk about my experiences then typed my words and rehearsed me. It's a long story but I gained confidence and have spoken in the Dominican Republic, Rome, Beirut and up and down the UK and Southern Ireland.

I helped to set up the Scottish Dementia Working Group, which is run for and by people with dementia in Scotland. This group is now widely consulted by authorities in Scotland and is respected for the quality of its members.

Time has been good to me. Recent tests show I am deteriorating, but what else can you expect with a deteriorating illness? I believe that with being active in your community and stretching your brain, you stand a chance of slowing down the progression, even though dementia always wins in the end. What have you to lose by trying it?

I meet so many lovely people, both people with dementia and support workers, that I lead an enriched and fruitful life.

I have my problems but I also have advantages.

Time to stop

Jane Gilliard & Mary Marshall

In this closing chapter we want to share some reflections on the contributions we received. We have found the whole process inspiring, thought provoking and often moving. We hope you share this experience. We feel that what started off as a relatively simple exercise has instead resulted in a most unusual and potentially transformational collection.

We started, as we said in our introduction, with the intention of raising awareness of the use of the word 'time' in dementia care. It is often used negatively, in a way that diminishes people with dementia. Yet most people who use the word in this way would have no intention of doing this. We think the book has achieved our objective, but it has also done a great deal more. Our contributors, all of whom are experts in dementia care, have taken the word and provided an extraordinarily rich tapestry of ideas, analysis, emotions, memories and reflections.

We thought people would take some usage of the word – such as 'no time for' or 'time pressure' and would share their experiences and views. Instead, they have taken off in all sorts of directions, sometimes in very personal and often unexpected ways. Our strongest impression is that it is time to really make time for people with dementia. In much the same way as the slow movement (www.slowmove-ment.com) is suggesting we slow down, many of our contributors are suggesting that we can be in the moment with people with dementia and that we will benefit from doing this. Our contributors are not hectoring us to try harder, but are rather saying that it is pleasurable and rewarding to join the world of people with dementia which is so strongly focused on the here and now. It is good for us and maybe good

for them. Christian Müller-Hergl (p81) warns us that the present may not always be a happy time for someone with dementia. Stephen Judd (p76) makes the wry observation that he may have to wait until he gets dementia to be able to slow down and enjoy the present.

Some of our contributors have suggested that it does not take any longer. Our parallel universe of time watching and rushing about can be compatible with the slower and timeless world of people with dementia if we do things differently. Eva Götell (p50), for example, suggests that we can care more effectively if we sing while we work. Other contributors have pointed out that people with dementia do not have unlimited time; it is a progressive disease. If we want to relish being in the moment with people with dementia, we should not put it off.

We have been surprised that so many of our contributors have written poetry in order to express their response to the words 'time and dementia'. We have also been surprised and moved at the numbers of people who chose to write about their own personal experience. We are sure that our readers will share with us our appreciation of this willingness to be open about personal pain and anxieties as well as happy stories of a meeting of minds.

Interestingly and perhaps unexpectedly, we get the impression that Eastern religions have a lot to offer with their focus on the present – for example, the Buddhist principle of living in the moment (see Andy Barker, p123, and Kate Allan, p82). Certainly the Protestant ethic's preoccupation with being busy now for a reward in the future is not really a helpful way to bridge the gap between the world of timetables and schedules and the world where time is of little consequence. As Muriel Weyl

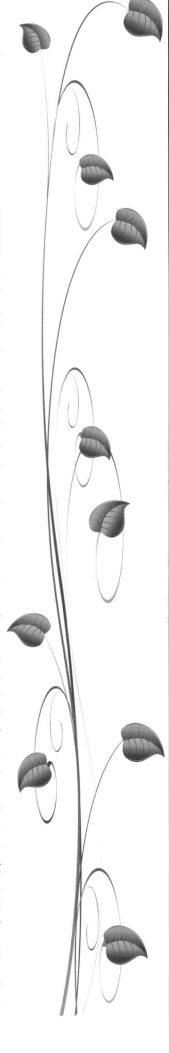

(2009) has written, "Peter may not be able to remember the time but he always has the time, time to read books, more than 50 of which are stacked in piles beside him, time to help me with whatever I need, time in which he doesn't worry about having time. He cannot understand why I rush around, why I worry about time, why my time is in deficit when his is in bounty." It is this notion of parallel universes which emerges strongly and which some contributors have sought to express in poetry. The question is, whose problem is it? The answer has to be that it is ours. It is our responsibility to make time.

One of our aspirations in editing this book is that we would have some impact on practice, or at least on helping people pause and reflect on their use of the word 'time'. It has struck us on reading the contributions that we might also have an impact on the direction of some developments in dementia care. We can see, for example, as yet unrealised potential in body clocks (see Ricky and Annie Pollock, p58). We need to know more about the difference it makes if the care plan matches the individual's diurnal rhythm, since the general under-standing seems to be that we all perform a lot more effectively if we do things at the right time for us.

We also wonder if there is potential in providing chiming clocks in people's houses and in care homes. We think there is definitely potential in more training programmes emphasising the skills of being in the moment, and of Indian Stretchable Time (Louise McCabe, p25). We think there might be merit in training programmes asking participants to write poetry as a way of tapping into empathy which may not be expressed in normal verbal commentary. We may need to think more about nature and dementia since the poems in this book use a lot of imagery from nature. There is certainly a need for us all to talk more about the gift of time that people with dementia bring us and how we recognise this and use it, which is really hard in a time-obsessed culture as Dave Anderson emphasises (p88).

We realise that some key areas relating to time and dementia have not been covered by the contributors to this book or have not been covered adequately. One is the need carers have for time – time for themselves, time for conversations, time for reflection and renewal, time to sleep properly and so on. Another is the time needed for a diagnosis and whether diagnosis is an event or a process. The same must be true of sharing the diagnosis. It is rarely satisfactory to do this once; indeed most people

with dementia and their carers seem to think it takes time to sink in and they often need to have the information repeated. Time for a single shared assessment is another key issue. How do we inform managers and planners who do not know enough about dementia that it can be a time-consuming process and certainly not something that is done in one visit? For a start, people with dementia will always tell you that their condition and competence varies from day to day. There is no denying that working with people with dementia takes more time than working with people who have not. Our contributors such as David Gribble (p41) have suggested that time taken to get to know people with dementia initially saves time later.

On a more prosaic note, the contributions made us revisit disability theory. We have both invested a lot of our career time in encouraging people to see the relevance of the disability approach (Oliver 1990) to dementia care. This crudely suggests that people have impairments (to their mobility, eyesight, cognition etc) but it is society which disables them. It is partly stigma. It is also lack of empathy and action about physical design, communica-tion and so on. We found ourselves thinking that attitudes to time are another way we disable people with some sorts of disability, especially of cognition. We expect them to function in our world and when they fail, we label them as incompetent. Instead we need to recognise that it is our responsibility to change the way we behave. We should not expect people with dementia to know the date, for example. We have always found that it is very difficult to get the disability movement to take on cognitive impairment, especially in older people. It does require a bit of lateral thinking but the principles apply in the same way. We have to make our world less disabling for people with the impairments of dementia, and one way to do this is to change some of our attitudes to time.

In conclusion, we want to emphasise that there is a lot of enjoyment to be had in being in the moment with people with dementia. They have the gift of time which we can accept and share. We could learn to make the most of the time we have and to enjoy everyday events and relationships more. We hope this book inspires people in dementia care take the time for themselves as well as for people with dementia.

Oliver M (1990) *The Politics of Disablement*. Macmillan, Basingstoke.
Weyl M (2009) Love song at the end of the day: a wife's journey. *Dementia* Vol 8, no 1, p 12.